I WANT TO BE
A SEAL TEAM MEMBER,

I WANT TO SWIM
THE DEEP BLUE SEA.

I WANT TO LIVE
A LIFE OF DANGER,

PICK UP YOUR SWIM FINS
AND RUN WITH ME!

TRADITIONAL NAVY SEAL RUNNING CADENCE

D1016384

Purchased from
Multnomah County Library
Title Wave Used Bookstore
216 NE Knott St, Portland, OR
503-988-5021

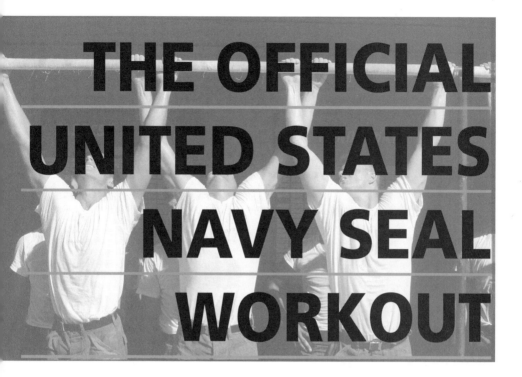

THE OFFICIAL UNITED STATES NAVY SEAL WORKOUT

RESEARCHED BY
ANDREW FLACH

PHOTOGRAPHED BY
PETER FIELD PECK

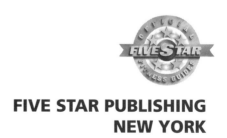

FIVE STAR PUBLISHING
NEW YORK

The Official United States Navy SEAL Workout
A Hatherleigh Press/Getfitnow.com Book

© 1998, 2003 by Andrew Flach
All rights reserved. No part of this book may be reproduced in any form or
by any means, electronic or mechanical, including photocopying, recording,
or by any information storage and retrieval system, without permission in
writing from the publisher.

Hatherleigh Press/Getfitnow.com Books
An Affiliate of W.W. Norton and Company, Inc.
5-22 46th Avenue, Suite 200
Long Island City, NY 11101
Toll Free 1-800-528-2550
Visit our Web sites getfitnow.com and hatherleighpress.com

Library of Congress Cataloging-in-Publication Data
Available upon Request

Cover design by Gary Szczecina
Text design and composition by DC Designs
Photographed by Peter Field Peck
with Cannon® cameras and lenses on Fuji® print and slide film
except photographs as noted: pages 11, 15, 16, 17, 21, 22 (bottom), 24, 56

Printed in Canada on acid-free paper
10 9 8 7 6 5 4 3 2 1

YOU MAY *THINK* YOU'RE PHYSICALLY FIT NOW. BUT CAN YOU:

1. Swim 500 yards using breast and/or sidestroke in 12 minutes and 30 seconds, rest for 10 minutes, then
2. Do 42 pushups in two minutes, rest for two minutes, then
3. Do 50 situps in two minutes, rest for two minutes, then
4. Do eight pull-ups, rest for 10 minutes, then
5. Run 1.5 miles wearing boots and pants in 11 minutes and 30 seconds?

If you can, consider this: Those are just the requirements to get into Navy SEAL training—*before* the actual training begins! If you can't do the above, you'll be able to—no sweat—by the time you master the workout program described in this book. That's because the Navy SEAL workout is part of the actual SEAL training regime. Whether you want to be a SEAL or just be as physically fit as the most extensively trained combat force in the world, this program can help you achieve your goal.

ACKNOWLEDGMENTS

Thanks to the staff of the offices listed below for their contributions, which helped to make this book possible.

Navy Office of Information
Pentagon, Washington, DC

Special thanks to:
RADM Kendell Pease
Chief of Information

LT Wendy Snyder
Public Affairs Officer

Naval Special Warfare Center
Coronado, CA

Special thanks to:
RADM Thomas Richards
Commanding Officer

LCDR James Fallin
Public Affairs Officer

BM2 Kevin Blake
BUD/S Instructor

Our editorial team: Heather Ogilvie and Susan Ruszala
Our design and production team:
Dede Cummings, Matt Sharff, and Gary Szczecina.
Our logistics and support team: Kevin Moran and Bruce Slagle.
And to the many others who contributed to the
success of this mission:
Thank you!

DEDICATION

To the gallant Frogmen
and SEALs, past and
present. You are our
nation's finest. You have
served heroically. May
this book inspire others
to follow you to glory!

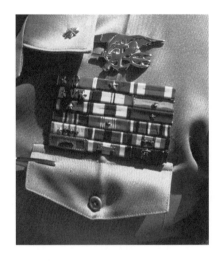

CONTENTS

PART I

PART II PHYSICAL TRAINING

Part III O' COURSE

PART IV GETTING READY

ABOUT THE SERIES

The Official Five Star Fitness Guides are designed to provide a fresh new perspective on the subject of personal health and fitness by documenting the physical training regimens of the United States Armed Forces.

To bring you this exciting information, we have shouldered our gear in the hot midday sun, on cold frosty mornings, in the dark of night. No workouts and training schedules were reorganized to meet our needs. Nor did we ask. We wanted to bring to you what's REAL. I like to think of these books as "fitness documentaries"—because that's what they are!

We have talked extensively with many individuals responsible for the physical fitness and welfare of the men and women of America's Armed Forces. We have discovered the most powerful workout and physical training routines in the world. We bring them to you with the hope that you will be inspired to value your health and pursue fitness activities throughout your life.

Wherever possible, primary source material is utilized. Documentation, interviews, briefs—all were assembled and culled for details and insights.

One important note: These books are not designed to be follow-to-the-letter workouts. That was never our intention. These books are a collection of information on the subject of fitness and physical training in the US military, full of techniques, routines, hints, suggestions and tips you can learn from. Your workout should be individualized. We highly recommend you review your fitness plan with a certified trainer, coach, or other individual who possesses the proper knowledge to advise you in such a manner. And of course, consult your physician before commencing any new fitness program or before you intensify your current regimen.

Good luck and may lifelong fitness be your goal!

Andrew Flach
Peter Field Peck

INTRODUCTION

How does one best describe the experience of witnessing Navy SEAL physical training? Do you write about the hot Southern California sun, the cloudless blue sky, the pounding surf ? Do you speak of the nonstop continuous training, the buzz of activity, the community of fitness? The seemingly countless pushups, pull-ups, situps, runs, and swims that each BUD/S student must perform if he is to become a Navy SEAL? Or do you speak of the men?

Quite honestly, the men I met that day at the Naval Special Warfare Center were a breed apart. The officers and instructors were exceptionally courteous. They were extremely knowledgeable and were eager to share their fitness information with me.

We met two BUD/S students when we needed to photograph the Navy SEAL Obstacle Course in action. They were among the most fit individuals I have seen. They ran the course flawlessly while Peter Peck photographed them tackling each obstacle. Many times Peter had to ask them repeat the obstacle so he could get a better camera angle to show important details. They obliged willingly, effortlessly. These two men were shining examples of America's youth: motivated, friendly, self-disciplined. Real role models.

When we arrived at the Naval Special Warfare Center the morning of our visit, August 18th, 1997, we were greeted by LCDR James Fallin, Public Affairs Officer. Commander Fallin advised Peter and me: "Be safe, have fun, and most importantly, tell the truth." I believe you'll find we accomplished all of those objectives, sir.

Enjoy this rare visit with our nation's elite US Navy SEALs.

Andrew Flach

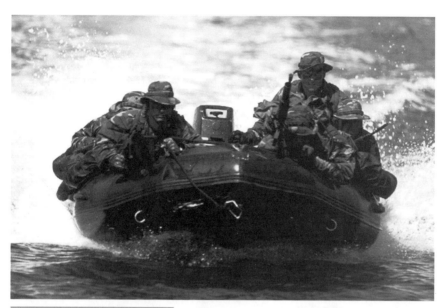

WHO ARE THE NAVY SEALS?

The SEALs are highly trained specialists that number less than one percent of the entire Navy. They are among the most elite fighting forces in the world, carrying out specialized missions that no other military unit can perform. The SEALs are extensively organized, trained, and equipped to conduct special operations, unconventional warfare, foreign internal defense, and clandestine operations in maritime and riverine environments. They are deployed worldwide, at a moment's notice, to support fleet and national operations. SEAL and SEAL Delivery Vehicle (SDV) Teams and Special Boat Units constitute the elite combat units of Naval Special Warfare. The extensive range of services and the outstanding combat record earn Naval Special Warfare a highly respected and revered reputation.

HISTORY OF THE SEALS

The history of the SEAL Teams dates back to 1943 when the first group of volunteers cleared obstacles from beaches chosen for amphibious landings during World War II. Though not yet known formally as SEALs, the volunteers in this mission constituted the first formal training of the Naval Combat Demolition Units (NCDUs). The NCDUs earned a distinguished reputation at Utah and Omaha beaches in Normandy and in Southern France and throughout the Pacific.

After World War II, the Navy organized its first underwater offensive strike teams and the NCDUs were consolidated into Underwater Demolition Teams (UDTs). UDTs were deployed to Korea, where beginning in 1950 they saw combat at Inchon, Wonsan, Iwon, and Chinnampo and used guerrilla warfare. The UDT's missions included demolition raids on bridges and tunnels accessible from the water. In addition, they also conducted limited minesweeping operations in harbors and rivers.

UNCONVENTIONAL FIGHTERS

The perilous political climate of the 1960s prompted Secretary of Defense Robert McNamara to call for new ideas on counter-aggression. Later recommendations by the Unconventional Activities Committee emphasized use of assault landing, reconnaissance, patrolling, transport of troops and supplies, fire support, air support, and the infiltration and exfiltration of personnel. In addition, the committee recommended the increased study of mine warfare and guerrilla warfare functions. The proposal noted the formation of SEAL Teams, an acronym of sea, air and land teams, having a universal and extensive training in guerrilla warfare. SEAL units were further defined as having a specialized capability for special operations in rivers, bays, harbors, canals, and estuaries. The missions of these units were either overt or covert and the units were to attack enemy shipping and land men and matèriel on hostile shores.

In 1962, the first SEAL teams were commissioned to conduct unconventional warfare, counter-guerrilla warfare, and clandestine operations in both blue- and brown-water envi-

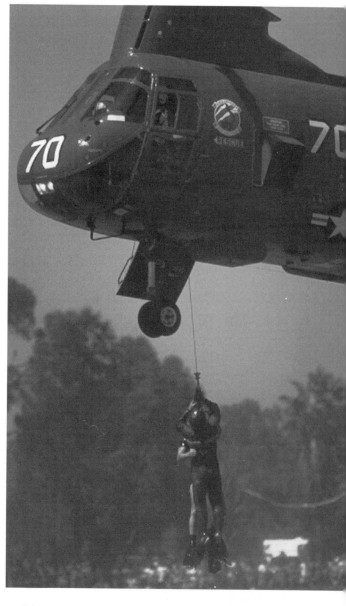

ronments. The Navy used former UDT forces to form these teams. The two teams formed were SEAL Team ONE on the West Coast and SEAL Team TWO on the East Coast. From 1962 to 1963, the Navy began to refine the basic structure for counterinsurgency warfare. The SEALs, along with other specialized units, became

PRE-BUD/S SCHOOLS

If you are interested in becoming a SEAL, the Naval Special Warfare BUD/S selection course provides an overview of SEAL Training and the Naval Special Warfare Community. The five-day course is offered to all active-duty Navy enlisted personnel from the Fleet, Service Schools, and Boot Camp. It is held at the Naval Training Command, Great Lakes. Applicants are temporarily assigned from their parent command to the selection course. The requirements for the course are the same as for BUD/S training. For further information, contact the Physical Training Rehabilitation Remediation office at (619) 437-0861 (DSN 577-0861).

the core of these highly specialized teams throughout the Vietnam War, where they compiled a successful record of combat missions.

THE SEALS TODAY

The changing face of world politics has created an even larger demand for the expansion of the SEAL teams since the close of the Vietnam War. The SEALs have recently conducted missions in Bosnia, Liberia, and the Persian Gulf. The SEALs have expanded in both size and capability, using former UDTs that have been redesignated as SEAL or SEAL Delivery Vehicle (SDV) Teams. Although the newly designated SEAL Teams acquired the SEAL mission, they retained the amphibious support mission inherited from the roots of the UDTs.

Today the SEALs are one of the country's most decorated combat units. Collectively, they have earned three Medals of Honor, numerous Navy Crosses, Legions of Merit, and Silver Stars, among hundreds of other medals.

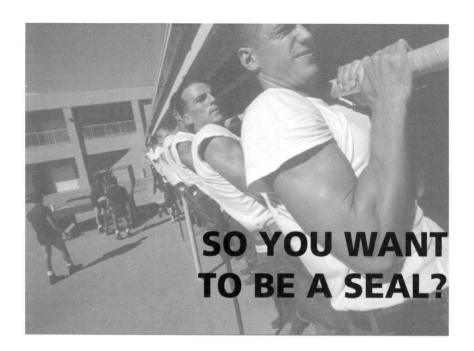

SO YOU WANT TO BE A SEAL?

Many experts consider Navy SEAL training to be the toughest military training in the world. It's a challenging program that pushes men to their physical and mental limits. Here's how it begins.

The intense training is a continual process that begins at BUD/S (Basic Underwater Demolition/SEAL) in Coronado, California. BUD/S requires each participant to be self-motivated and physically fit. In addition to the physical training to improve stamina and strength, BUD/S tests your leadership ability as well. There is no room for substandard performance—at BUD/S your personal best is required every minute of every day. A regimented diet, exercise, and positive attitude are essential for success and a rewarding experience. The workouts in this book will help prepare you for the physical stress of the extremely thorough training program at BUD/S.

There are three Phases of training at BUD/S, described below.

FIRST PHASE: BASIC CONDITIONING.

First Phase consists of basic conditioning. The duration of First

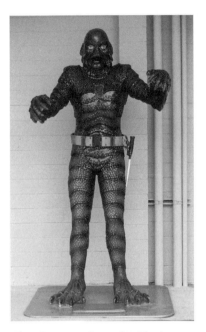

The Creature from the Black Lagoon, a gift from BUD/S Class 62, is located in the central courtyard of the BUD/S training center.

Phase is eight weeks. The physical conditioning consists of running, swimming, and calisthenics, and grows more difficult as the weeks progress. Students are required to participate in weekly four-mile timed runs in boots, timed obstacle courses, and swim distances up to two miles wearing fins in the ocean. They also learn small boat seamanship.

The fifth week of First Phase is called "Hell Week." During Hell Week, there are five and a half days of continuous training with a maximum of four hours of sleep. This week is designed to test the individual's physical and mental motivation while still in First Phase and relies heavily on teamwork. The last three weeks of First Phase teach methods of conducting hydrographic surveys and how to prepare a hydrographic chart.

SECOND PHASE: DIVING.

The successful completion of First Phase proves that you are ready for more serious training. Second Phase concentrates on combat Self Contained Underwater Breathing Apparatus (SCUBA). The diving skills you learn during this seven-week period train you in the skills that separate SEALs from all other Special Operations forces. Although the physical training used in First Phase continues, students must complete the four-mile runs, two-mile swims, and obstacle course in less time. Students concentrate on two types of SCUBA: open circuit (compressed air) and closed circuit

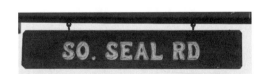

(100 percent oxygen). The ultimate goal is to train the student with basic combat swimmer skills to qualify as a combat diver. Again, a progressive dive schedule is used to emphasize the basic combat skills needed in order to qualify as a combat diver.

THIRD PHASE: LAND WARFARE.

This is a physically intense ten-week training phase with the focus on demolition, reconnaissance, weapons, and tactics. Students learn land navigation, small-unit tactics, rappelling, military land and underwater explosives, and weapons training. In addition, the run distances increase and the minimum passing times are once again lowered for the runs, swims, and obstacle course. Students apply techniques learned in the training program during the final four weeks on San Clemente Island in California.

After graduation from BUD/S, there is additional training. Before reporting to their first Naval Special Warfare Command, graduates receive three weeks of basic parachute training at the Army Airborne School, Fort Benning, Georgia. Navy corpsmen who

ARE YOU NAVY SEAL MATERIAL?

In addition to passing a physical screening test to enter the Navy's SEAL training (known as BUD/S), you must also meet these general requirements:

1. Pass a diving physical exam
2. Pass an eye exam—eyesight cannot be worse than 20/40 in one eye and 20/70 in the other eye and must be correctable to 20/20 with no color blindness
3. Minimum ASVAB score: VE + AR = 104, MC = 504.
4. Be 28 years old or younger
5. Be male

If you meet these requirements, start planning your Navy career today. Call your local Navy recruiter. Start the workout program immediately—with motivation, you can incorporate these exercises into a busy high school or college schedule.

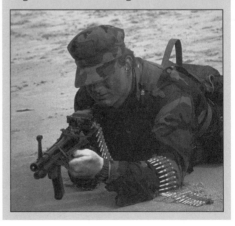

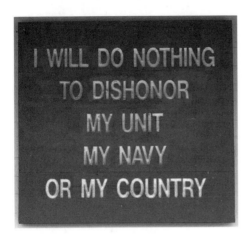

I WILL DO NOTHING
TO DISHONOR
MY UNIT
MY NAVY
OR MY COUNTRY

complete BUD/S and Basic Airborne Training also attend two weeks of Special Operations Technicians Training at the Naval Special Warfare Center, Colorado. In addition, they participate in a 30-week course of instruction in diving medicine and medical skills called 18-D (Special Operations Medical Sergeant Course). During this time, students receive training in burns, gunshot wounds, and trauma.

Qualified personnel are awarded a SEAL Naval Enlisted Classification (NEC) Code and Naval Special Warfare Insignia after the successful completion of a six-month probationary period with a Team. New combat swimmers serve the remainder of their first enlistment (two and a half to three years) in either a SEAL Delivery Vehicle (SDV) or SEAL Team. Upon re-enlistment, members may be ordered to additional training and another SDV or SEAL Command where they will complete the remainder of a five-year sea tour. Advanced courses include Sniper, Diving Supervisor, language training, and SEAL Tactical Communications. There are also shore duty opportunities available in research and development as well as instructor duty and overseas assignments.

For information about becoming a Navy SEAL, see the Recruitment Information in the back of the book.

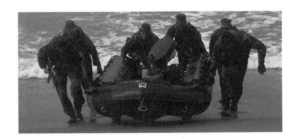

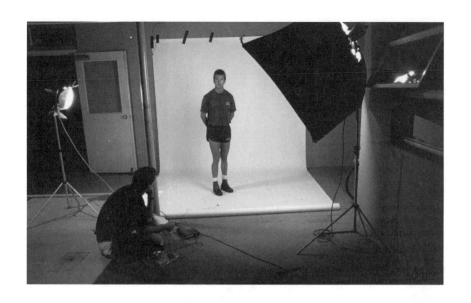

MEET BM2 KEVIN BLAKE,
NAVY SEAL INSTRUCTOR

We were fortunate to have an experienced BUD/S instructor, BM2 Kevin Blake, share his fitness knowledge with us during our visit to the Naval Special Warfare Center. Kevin demonstrated the stretching and PT exercises for us, as well as providing insight into SEAL training in all Phases of BUD/S.

Kevin has been a Navy SEAL for almost 15 years. Since 1982, he has been a member of SEAL Team 2, SEAL Team 3, and SEAL Team 5. As a Navy SEAL, Kevin has served in Europe, the Mediterranean, Southeast and Southwest Asia, and the Western Pacific. In addition, Kevin spent a year in Kodiak, Alaska, as a Winter Warfare Instructor. In his spare time, Kevin is an avid rock climber, cyclist, and triathlete.

Kevin is currently asssigned as Fourth Phase BUD/S instructor. Fourth Phase is a special pre-training Phase, and precedes First Phase. It is called Fourth Phase because it is the newest Phase of BUD/S to be developed. Fourth Phase concentrates heavily on physical conditioning and was designed to help BUD/S candidates ready themselves to enter First Phase.

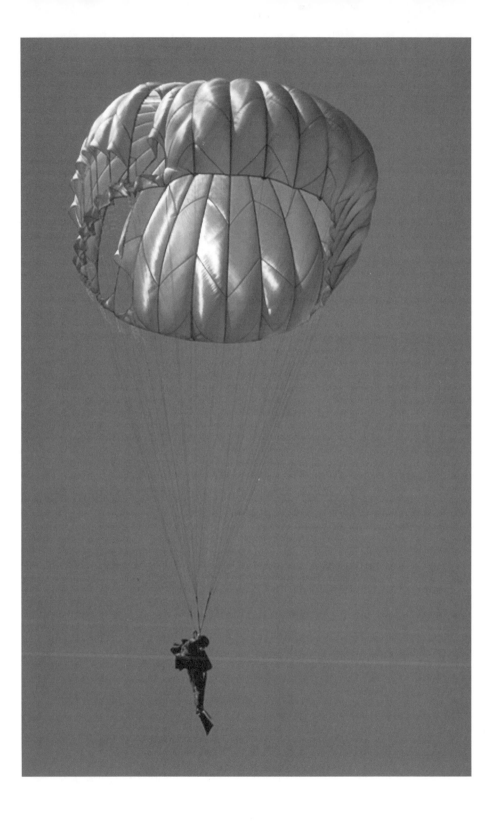

STAYING MOTIVATED

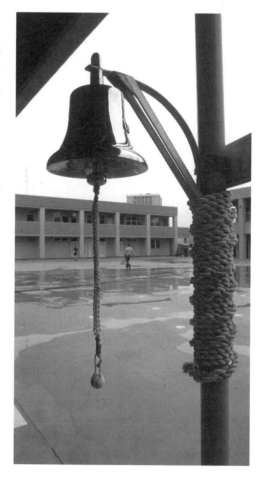

A BUD/S student's most valuable motivation comes from his brothers-in-training. The BUD/S class pulls together. Unique about SEAL training is the pressure and stress on the students — which they sometimes can perceive as a negative — but the students do have a positive source to tap into.

Tradition has it that if a BUD/S student decides to drop from training, he must ring The Bell three times and place his helmet on the ground beneath it. This gesture is repeated many times during a BUD/S class. The dropout rate can be as high as 75% or greater.

They develop spirit as a class of men going through something that's demanding, challenging, and desirable.

An infectious spirit develops within the class, especially as SEALs go through training and come closer to the end. They start to gel as a class—you can really see and feel the motivation.

But what if you're not a BUD/S student, and maybe you're interested in being a SEAL someday, thinking about going to BUD/S, and working out at home to get yourself in shape? What then? What can you do to stay motivated? Find somebody to be a support person—someone who shares your dreams and goals and values. You can help each other to stay motivated, and by training together you'll get awesome results!

Positive mental imagery is also important. Have a clear idea of your goal. Keep focused on that image. Keep thinking of it. Make it a positive mental image of who, what, and where you want to be and then go for it! Self-motivation is a powerful tool.

Here's one example to make your training more effective. Let's say you're running down the beach or road. Think of yourself as being in a race. Think of the road as being lined with people who are cheering for you. You'll notice your form getting better— you'll run faster, harder. Next thing you know you're done! You've had a great workout using positive mental imaging as a self-inspirational tool.

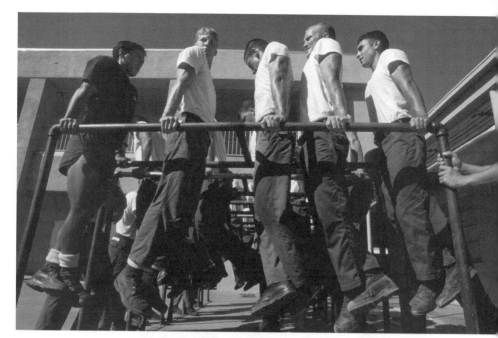

STRETCHES

INTRODUCTION

Stretching is often the warmup for exercise programs, but SEALs prefer to warm up *before* they start to stretch. If you go right into stretching cold, it's not only painful but it can be injurious too. You might want to take an easy run, say two or three miles and then stretch. At that point you will be warmed up and ready to go. Stretch—and *then* get into the workout. If you don't have the time to run first, try a 15-minute fast walk, do jumping jacks, or perform any other calisthenics that get the blood pumping.

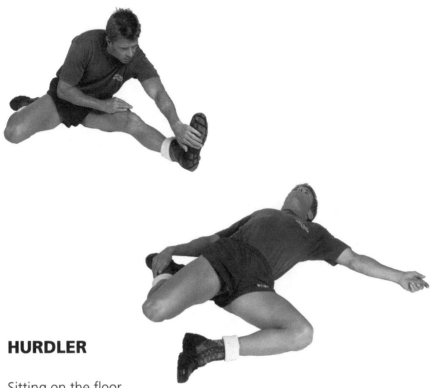

HURDLER

Sitting on the floor,
form a 90° angle with your legs as shown. Relax. Feel the weight go
down into your leg muscles and then gently lean forward without
bouncing. A little bit of pulsing is okay just to increase that stretch.
Reach out and grab the palm of your foot. Relax everything a little
more and just pull into it—not so it causes pain, but it should feel
good. You do not want to cause pain. Keep your back straight.
Eventually lie down on the leg. It takes a while—weeks and months
of stretching—before you attain maximum flexibility.

The second part of the Hurdler Stretch is to lie back and stretch out
as in the second photo. It's important to let your body go into a natural position, where everything is relaxed and you can concentrate on
the muscle that needs to be stretched. Hold for 30 seconds, then lean
over.

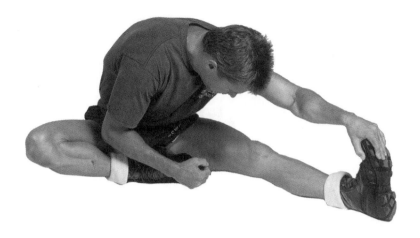

MODIFIED HURDLER

In the Modified Hurdler, bring your foot in as the photo shows. This stretch is easier on the back than the regular Hurdler, and it also helps stretch out the lower back. It's just as much of a lower back stretch as it is a hamstring stretch. Stretching out the lower back is important and becomes even more important as a person ages.

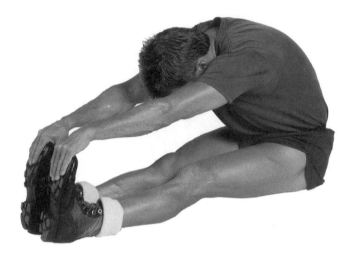

SITTING HEAD TO KNEE

The Sitting Head to Knee is a double hamstring stretch. Put both legs straight out. Grab the toes. This is another full back-of-the-leg stretch, from the calves to the buttocks. Hold and pull down gradually—not causing pain—and you might want to rock gently from side to side a little bit just to feel the stretch go around the sides of your legs.

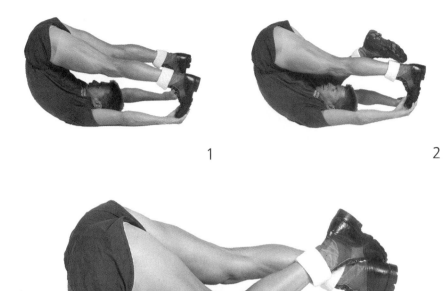

1

2

3

BACK ROLLERS

The Back Roller is a really good back and hamstring stretch. Relax and just let gravity pull you down. Then you can let go with one leg and cock your hips so that the hip that's connected to the leg that's being stretched helps stretch the back muscles down the length of your spine. Repeat the stretch on the other side.

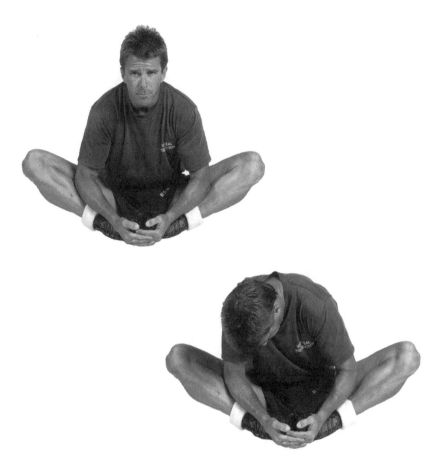

BUTTERFLY STRETCH

The Butterfly is a favorite. It's very relaxing. Just put both soles of your feet together and bring them in close. The point is to stretch the tendons and the ligaments in the groin. Get your feet in as close as you can, flat together, and then push down on your shins and calves with your elbows. Stretch with your neck and head down. You can also rock back and forth gently—nothing real drastic or jerky. This increases flexibility all the way around.

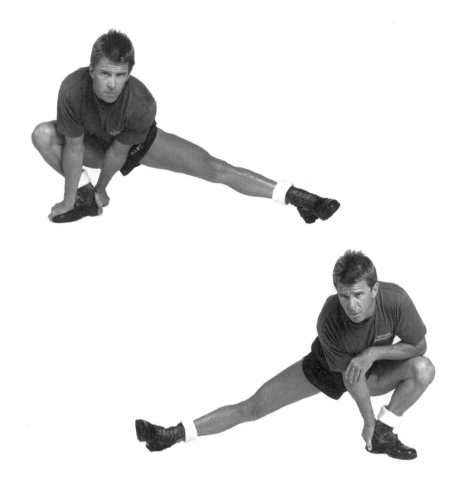

GROIN STRETCH

Stand with legs a little wider than shoulder length apart. The goal is to stretch your tendons from the inside of your thigh down to your knee. You might want to put a hand on your heel as shown. It provides support and it keeps your other leg down flat. Relax your body and lean into the stretch. Repeat on the other side.

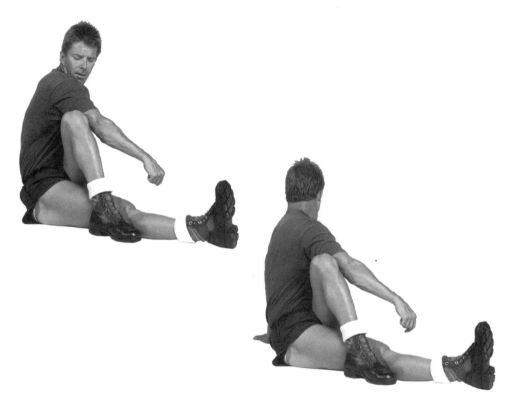

ILIO TIBIAL BAND STRETCH

To start, put your right leg out flat and cross your left leg over so that the outside of the heel is by the knee. The effective part of this stretch is putting your elbow on the outside of your crossed-over knee, pushing on it, and turning so you can feel the stretch all the way through the upper hamstrings, through the gluteal region, and into the lower back. Turn your head as you stretch. Repeat on the other side.

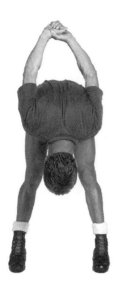

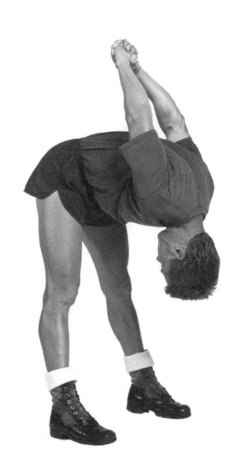

SWIMMER STRETCH

Bend over as shown, grabbing a wrist with one hand or interlocking your fingers, and then pull it back and gently stretch out the lats and the frontal deltoids. The Swimmer Stretch is something you might want to try with your workout buddy for maximum effectiveness, although it can be performed individually too.

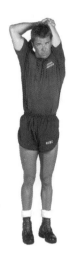

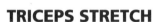

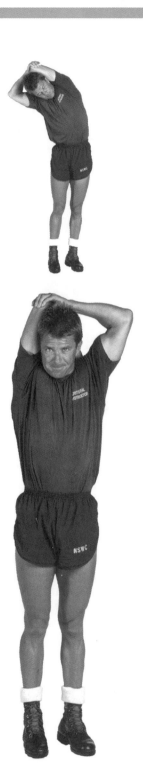

TRICEPS STRETCH

Put your right elbow up on the right side of the head, placing your right hand in the middle of your shoulder blades. Grab your right elbow with your other hand, and then pull it back, nice and easy, stretching your triceps. This can turn into a pretty good lat or side stretch if you bend to your left as shown. Reverse arm positions to stretch the other triceps and side.

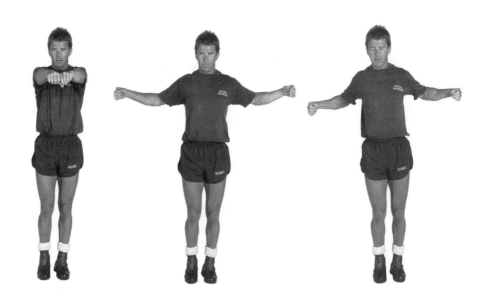

PRESS-PRESS-FLING

Press-Press-Fling starts out with your arms straight out front, horizontal. Then bring them back in a butterfly-like chest movement with your elbows bent at a 90° angle—snap it back to get the most range of motion. That's the Press. Do it twice. Press-Press. Be careful not to snap too hard. And avoid this stretch if you are recovering from a shoulder injury. The Fling is accomplished by opening your arms nice and wide and

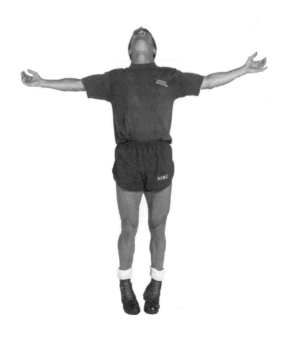

snapping back. At the same time, come up on your toes and arch your back. Press-Press-Fling. It's easier than it sounds.

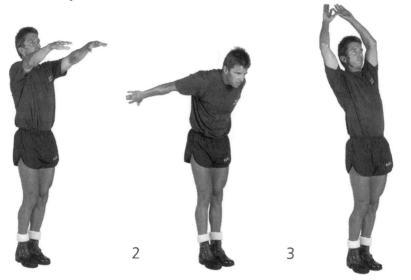

1   2   3

UP, BACK AND OVER

Up, Back and Over starts with both arms at your side. Lift your arms straight up. That's the Up. Then fling them behind you, like in the Swimmer's Stretch. That's the Back. Return to the starting position and then do a big reverse arm circle. Stretch it all the way around back to the starting position. That's the Over. Then repeat.

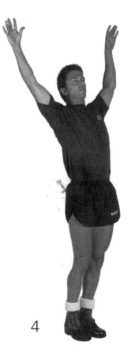

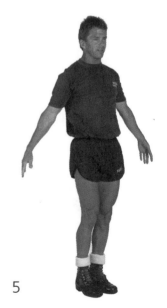

4   5

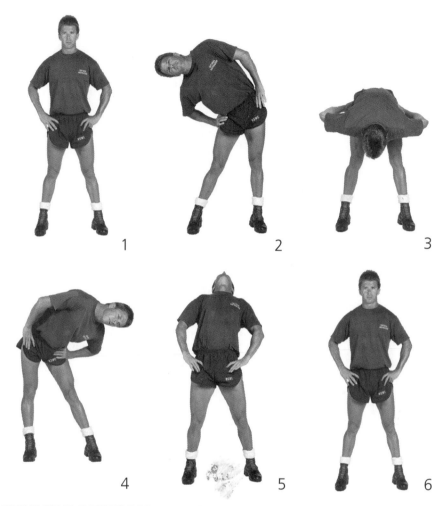

1   2   3

4   5   6

TRUNK ROTATION

Hands on your hips, feet about shoulder width apart. It should be a stable and comfortable stance. Starting off nice and slow, bend at your waist to the right side. Lean into it a bit. Return to the start position. Bend to the front. Return. Bend to the left. Return. Then bend to the back. And return. Half way through the desired number of repetitions, it is recommended that you reverse direction, starting to the left.

39

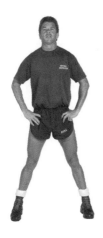

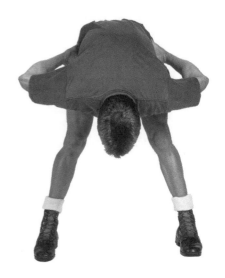

TRUNK BENDING FORE AND AFT

Trunk Bending Fore and Aft is pretty simple. Hands on your hips, feet about shoulder width apart. Bend to the Front. One. Return to the starting position. Two. Bend to the Rear. Three. Return. Four. As in all exercises, keep an even tempo as you count the repetitions. One, two, three, ONE. One, two, three, TWO. One, two, three, THREE. And so on. It keeps your mind clear so you can remember how many you've done. Or how many more you have to do!

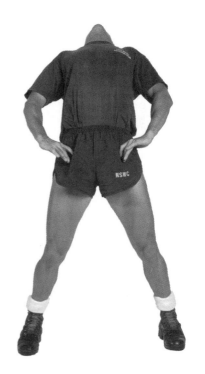

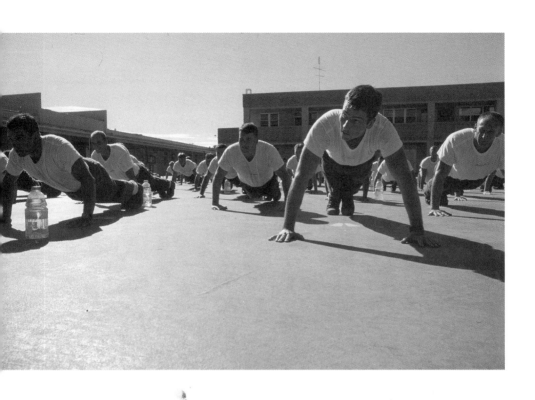

UPPER
BODY

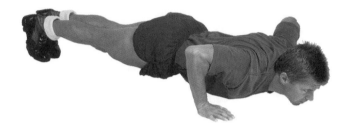

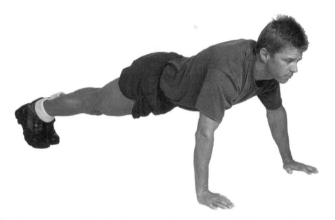

PUSHUPS

Everyone should be familiar with this standard physical training (PT) exercise. A Navy SEAL does many of these to get strong. Follow the instructions carefully 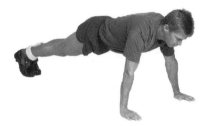 and focus on developing proper technique and soon you'll be cranking out hundreds of pushups. Starting position is shown in the top photo. Hands are a comfortable width apart—a little wider than the shoulders is typical. Have your feet together and lower yourself down to the deck leaving less than a fist's width of room between your chest and the ground. Keep your back perfectly straight—the SEALs emphasize a completely straight body when performing this classic pushup or its variations. Don't let your back sag or your body bend at the waist with your buttocks higher than your back. Not only does it look bad, you can hurt yourself in the process. Learn them and do them right!

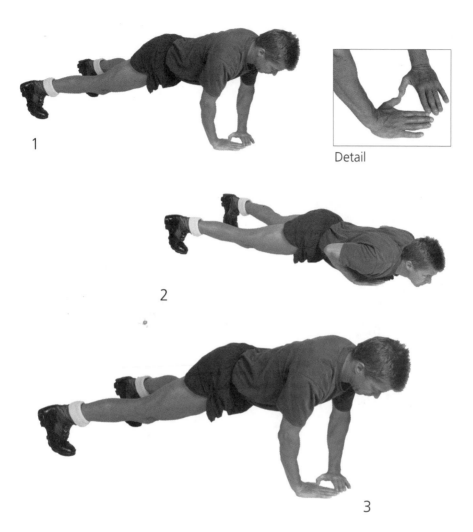

1

Detail

2

3

TRICEPS PUSHUPS

The Triceps Pushup is an excellent variation which focuses, naturally, on the triceps. Key to the Triceps Pushup is forming a small diamond with your thumbs and index fingers (see photo detail). For this pushup, spread your legs a couple of feet apart to enhance stability, and lower yourself so your chest meets your hands. Keep your back straight and feel the burn in your triceps.

43

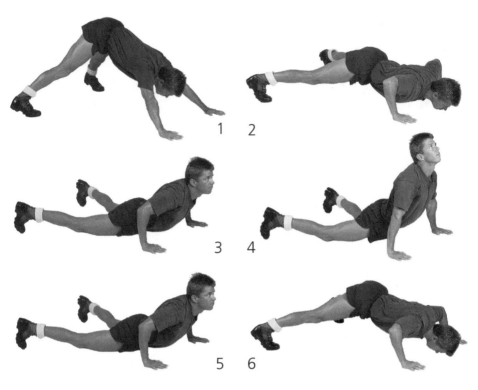

DIVE-BOMBER PUSHUPS

The Dive-Bomber Pushup is multi-dimensional: it incorporates declined, flat, and inclined press movements that you see at the gym

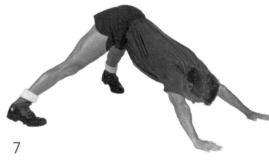

on those respective benches. Take a little bit wider set on the hands than on a regular pushup. Like the Triceps Pushup, keep your feet separated in back (about the same distance as the hands are up front). Lower yourself down, leading with your nose, almost scraping it on the deck at midpoint, then raise your whole body up as shown in the photo. Keep the movement smooth as you follow through. Reverse the motion all the way back to the starting position and repeat. And repeat. And repeat....

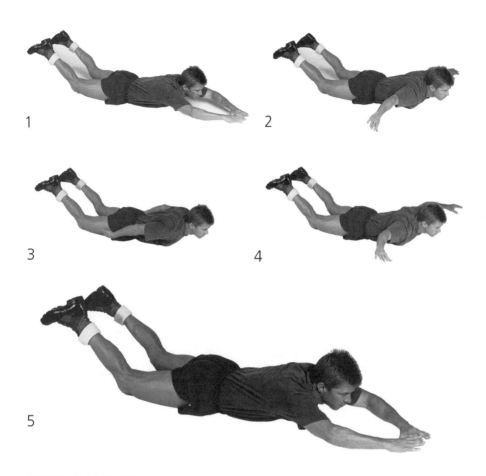

1

2

3

4

5

ARM HAULERS

These are good to add on at the end of the pushups series. Get down on your belly, feet and arms up off the deck so everything's arched, with your arms stretched out in front of the head. Following a full range of motion, sweep all the way back to the thighs and all the way forward again. Do it as a four-count exercise: one, two, three, ONE. One, two, three, TWO. One, two, three, THREE. The Arm Hauler is like a breaststroke on land. Keep it nice and slow—it's torture for the delts.

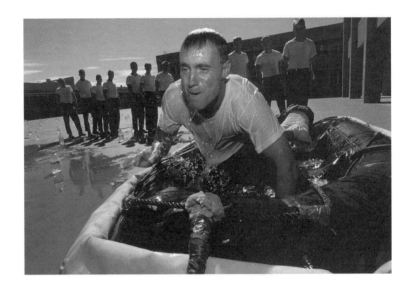

During Grinder PT sessions, SEAL candidates fill up one or two IBSs (INFLATABLE BOAT SMALL) with water. They do it for a couple of reasons. If a guy seems to be overheating they will send him to the IBS to cool off. They can even ask to do it if they want to—they can quickly douse themselves without having to run all the way out to the surf.

Sometimes, if a guy's not performing and needs a little motivation, the instructors send him to the IBS to help him reconsider his motivation. The water can get a little nasty after several dozen overheated BUD/S students go for a dunk. Take my word: Don't try this at home!

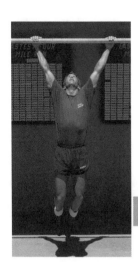

PULL-UPS
AND DIPS

What's the secret to the perfect pull-up?

Here are a few tips. Keep your back arched. Think of your arms as a set of hooks—try not to bring your biceps into play too much. Isolate your back. Pull-ups are a back movement, though your arms will inevitably get pumped. And don't forget to stretch.

Let's say you can do seven pull-ups, how are you going to do eight?

Here are two solid ways of cranking out more pull-ups: First, find a gym with a Lat Pull-Down machine and start adding weight up to 10 or 25 pounds more than your body weight and do five solid pull-downs. Then reduce the weight to 10 or 25 pounds below your body weight and go for eight or nine pull-downs. With this technique you're getting accustomed to doing more of the pull-up movement plus you're adding resistance. It will make you stronger to lift your own body weight when doing actual pull-ups.

A second way to increase your ability to perform proper Navy SEAL dead-hang pull-ups (and we mean this—no bicycling or kicking your legs to get up and over the bar) is to work out with a buddy. Your buddy can actually assist you by pushing upward on your hips or on your lower back as you do them, just enough to help you squeeze out a couple more on the pull-up bar.

Navy SEALs do many regular pull-ups and pull-up variations.

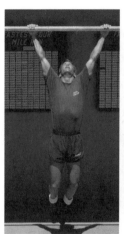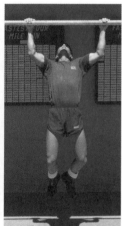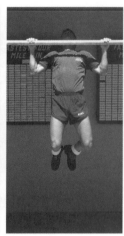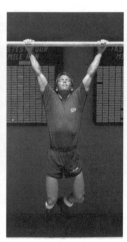

REGULAR GRIP

The regular grip pull-up is performed routinely. Grab the pull-up bar with your arms spaced a little wider than your shoulders. Keep your thumb and fingers on the same side of the bar. From a dead-hang, thinking of the arms as hooks, work your back, not your arms. Keep your back arched. Look up. Pull yourself up over the bar and lower yourself in a controlled fashion. Concentrate on utilizing proper technique for all of the pull-up variations. Form is key.

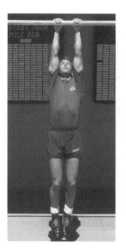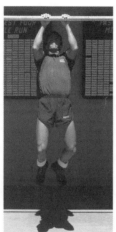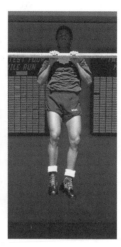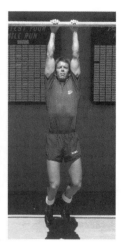

CLOSE GRIP

Grab the pull-up bar palms facing out, your hands a couple of inches apart. Same technique as in the regular grip pull-up. Back arched. Hands like hooks. Do them right. Notice in the photo the true dead-hang. There is absolutely no leg motion whatsoever. If you are having trouble keeping your legs still, or if you are on the tall side, you might want to bend your knees a bit and cross your legs at the ankles. This will increase your stability and will reduce the tendency to bicycle.

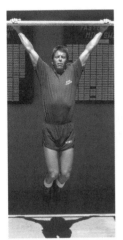 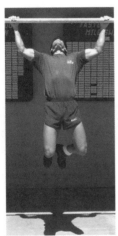 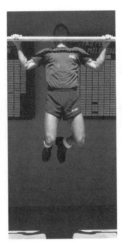 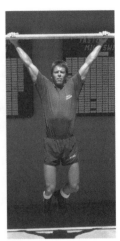

WIDE GRIP

Wide grip pull-ups are definitely challenging. Set your arms as wide as possible—but not so it's uncomfortable. The same technique applies: Hands like hooks. Use your back, and your deltoids get a great workout. Pull yourself up and lower yourself down. Nice and easy. Always in control.

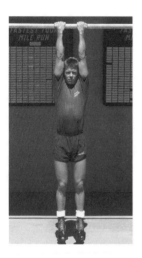 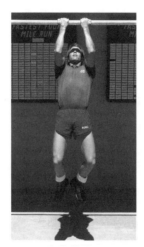 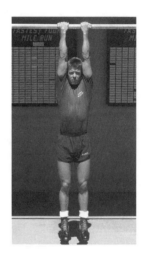

REVERSE GRIP

Otherwise known as the "chin-up" or "curls," reverse grip pull-ups are sometimes referred to as "curls for the girls." Not that they are easy, mind you. Especially after you have cranked out a total of 50 or 60 pull-up combinations in the hot sun.

Reverse grip pull-ups are performed exactly like the close-grip pull-ups, only you reverse your grip so your palms are facing toward you (again keeping fingers and thumbs on the same side of the bar). Set your hands a few inches apart and perform the exercise. You will find this pull-up variation uses more biceps strength than the others.

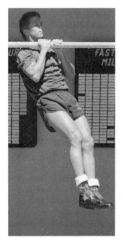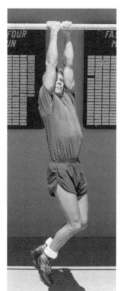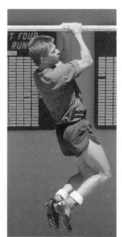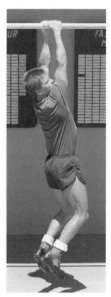

CLIFFHANGERS

The Cliffhanger is a challenging pull-up. It provides a multi-dimensional workout: biceps, delts, and lats all share in the fun. Start by standing directly underneath the pull-up bar and turn so your body is perpendicular to it. Grab the bar with your right hand and then grab the bar with your left hand, making certain that your left hand is furthest away from you. Make certain that both hands touch. Now pull yourself up, bringing your right shoulder to meet the bar, as shown in the photo. Lower yourself in a controlled manner. Do the exact same pull-up again. And again. When you are halfway through your set, switch your grip and do your Cliffhangers on the left side.

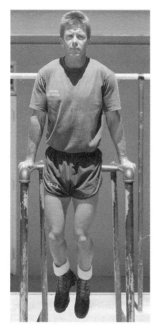
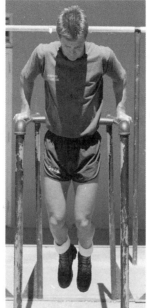
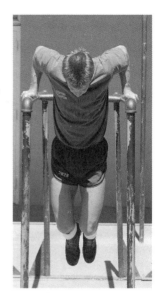

DIPS

Dips are another staple in Navy SEAL workouts. Proper form is essential. Your back should be kept straight and arched. Keep your elbows in. Thumbs facing forward. Lower yourself in a controlled manner until your elbows are just at a 90° angle. Don't bend further than 90°—it's an invitation for injury. Come up in smooth motion and avoid locking your elbows when at the starting position.

Workout Tip: If you want to work the chest more, look down and it will put more stress on the chest. If you want to work the triceps more, look up and you'll be working the triceps more.

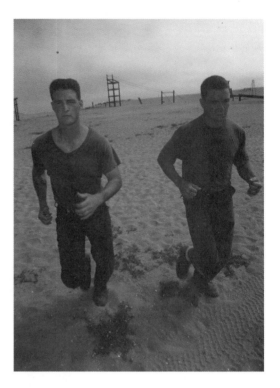

THE RUNNING PROGRAM

SEALs typically run three- to four-mile runs down the beach during training. Sometimes, depending on the tide and who's leading the run, they'll run down on the hard-packed sand at low tide or up on the soft sand, which makes for harder running. SEALs sprint on certain days. They also do "berm" runs: over the berm (which is like a sand dune), down to the water line, and turn around and run back over the berm again.

Long runs are great for building stamina. Sprints are essential for developing speed and strength.

"THE ONLY EASY DAY WAS YESTERDAY"

THE SWIMMING PROGRAM

Navy SEALs are water-borne warriors. Hence they do a lot of swimming. Their swims are varied to prepare them for combat mission swim conditions. Here's an example of a pool swim "evolution" designed to build strength and stamina.

The swim starts with a warmup of 800 to 1,000 meters using the "underwater recovery stroke" or SEAL combat swimmer stroke, which is a very aggressive form of the traditional sidestroke. After the

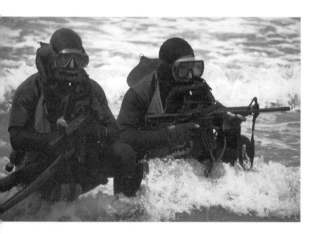

warmup they will do 50-meter swims on the minute, meaning a new swimmer departs every minute, and each swimmer is expected keep pace. It's a lot to expect for some people so the instructors inevitably break it into groups of slower and faster swimmers. The goal is to keep the 50 meters per minute pace.

They'll perform about ten of these relays and then go to 100m/1 min:20 sec. A swimmer will depart on a 100-meter swim every 1:20. This is performed for a specified number of repetitions, perhaps five or ten. Then they go to 200-meter relays—fewer repetitions, of course—with timed departures every 2:30. Just another easy day in the life of a Navy SEAL.

SEALs also routinely perform ocean swims, and learn drown-proofing techniques, underwater knot tying, open and closed circuit SCUBA, hydrographic reconnaissance, and other specialties depending upon the Phase of their training.

LOWER BODY

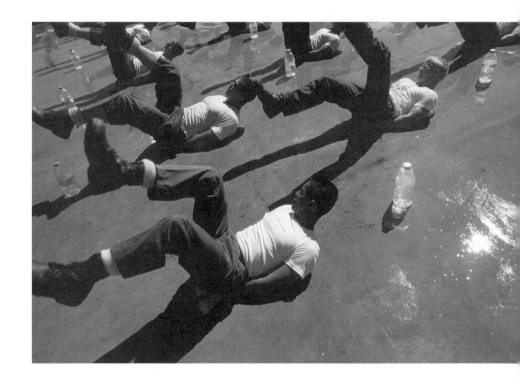

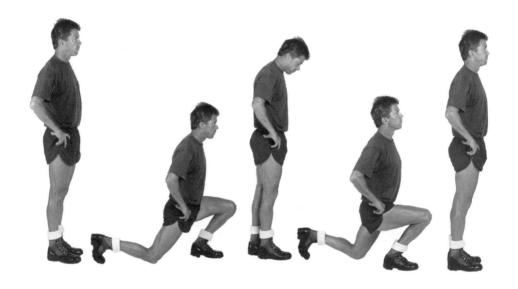

LUNGES

The importance of excellent leg strength to a Navy SEAL goes without saying. The first exercise is the Lunge. Start with your hands on your hips to get them out of the way. Some guys in the past have put their hands behind their head—this is not advisable as it pulls down on the neck, throwing you way out of form and risking injury. To perform a proper lunge keep your back straight and protected. This is not a down-up exercise. It is a step forward-down-up motion that is repeated again and again. Try these in reverse for fun (but look where you are going!).

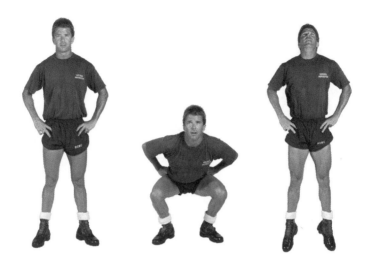

SQUAT LEAPS

A regular Squat is a down-up motion. What SEALs do to make it interesting is to turn it into a jump. This kind of explosive training is known as plyometrics. Plyometric training is used in many sports, such as basketball, where power and speed are required goals. Start with your feet about shoulder width apart, toes pointed out so your knees align properly to minimize injury risk. Now with your hands on your hips, lower yourself so your knees are bent to about a 90° angle. Then from this position, propel yourself upward as if a C-4 charge went off under the soles of your feet. Land safely and repeat.

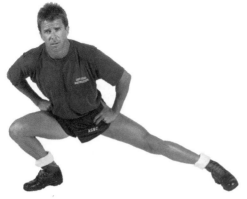

SIDE LUNGE

Although this looks like the Groin Stretch, it is performed differently. It's not a stretch, it's an exercise. Starting with your legs wider than shoulder width apart (as shown), lower yourself to the right by bending your right leg and shifting your weight to the right. Your knee should be just about 90°. Push up off your right foot and return to the start position. Now do the same on your left side. Repeat the exercise right-left-right-left.

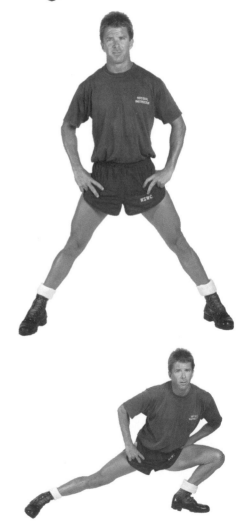

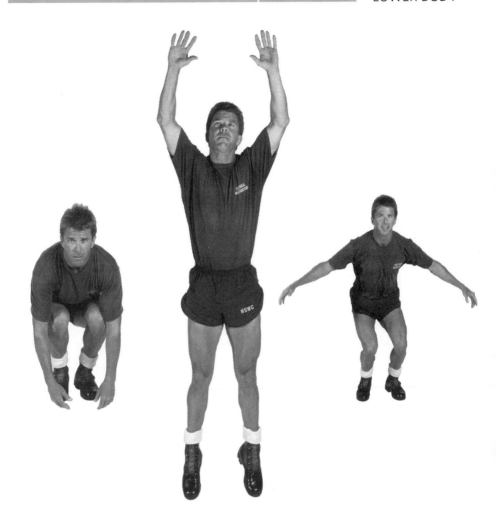

STAR JUMPERS

Another excellent plyometric.

Start in a squat position as shown. Now with a burst of energy, jump up with your hands high above your head. Grab a star while you're up there. After all, with the Navy SEALs *anything's* possible!

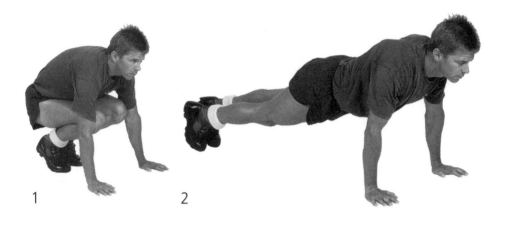

1   2

EIGHT-COUNT BODY BUILDER

The Eight-Count Body Builder is a Navy SEAL PT classic. It really is a unique exercise combining a variety of moves and muscles and the result is a powerful PT exercise that works the upper body, lower body, and cardiorespiratory system. Some might call it the mother of all pushups.

Here's how you do it. Begin in a standing position. Move to a squat position with your arms slightly more than shoulder width apart and count "1." Thrust your legs straight back, count "2." Keeping your back straight, lower yourself in a picture perfect pushup "3" and up "4." Kick your legs apart like a scissor "5" then kick them back together "6." Pull your legs back in a reverse thrust motion "7." And stand "8." You have just performed one Eight-Count Body Builder. Congratulations!

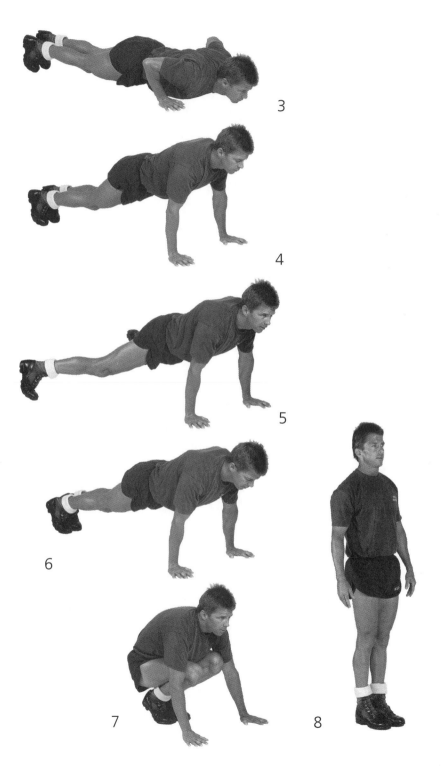

3

4

5

6

7

8

ABDOMINALS

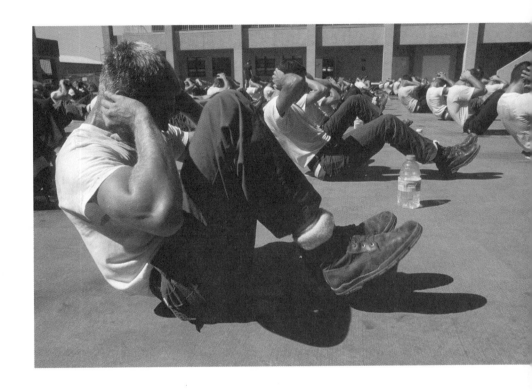

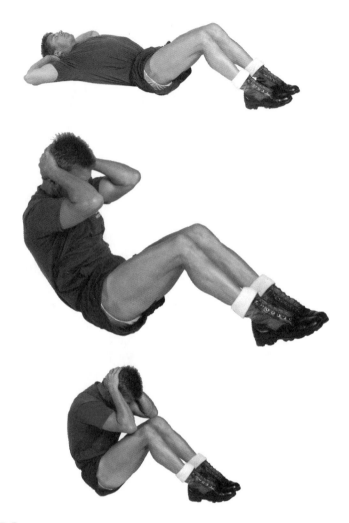

SITUPS

Another PT classic. Learn to do them right: start with knees bent, at a comfortable angle, hands clasped behind the head, elbows on the deck. Come up, touch your elbows to your thighs, and return. It's important to keep your back rounded. Guys who are not in good shape tend to arch the back—an injury invitation. So to reduce your risk, roll up and roll down, gently!

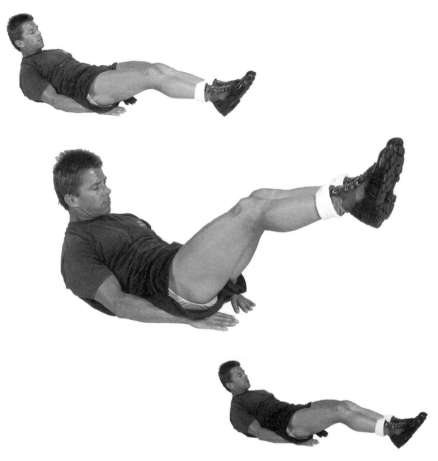

LEG LEVERS

Leg Levers are a lower abdominal exercise. To begin, take your hands and form a sort of "cradle" for your body (see photo). This arm position encourages the back to stay rounded —again to re-duce risk of injury or strain. With your back rounded on the ground, lift your feet about six inches off the ground. Don't lock your legs out straight; keep them a little flexed. Concentrate on using your lower abs and lift your legs from six inches up to maybe 26 or 30 inches, max. Repeat. Repeat. Repeat.

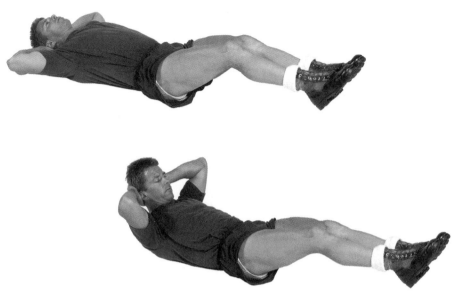

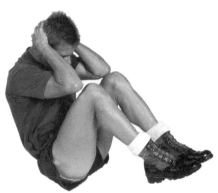

ATOMIC SITUPS

Welcome to the Nuclear Age! Why is it called an Atomic Situp? Well, after two cycles of 20 of these you'll feel like someone dropped an A-Bomb on your belly. Lie on your back and place your hands behind your head as shown. Extend your legs and lift your feet about six inches off the deck, keeping your legs slightly flexed. That's the starting position. Perform a situp while at the same time pulling your knees into your chest. It's a tough one, no doubt. Just keeping your balance is challenging.

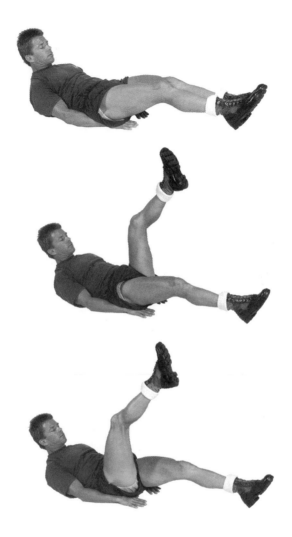

BACK FLUTTER KICKS

Navy SEALs do a lot of swimming. Back Flutter Kicks are a great way to strengthen your hip flexors—muscles used consistently during long ocean swims. Back Flutter Kicks are a traditional and staple PT exercise. SEALs do a lot of these. Starting position is the same as in Leg Levers. Start kicking. Keep your range of motion between six inches to 36 inches max. It's a four-count exercise. One, two, three, ONE. One, two, three, TWO. One, two, three, THREE. And so on.

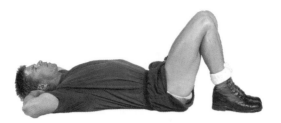

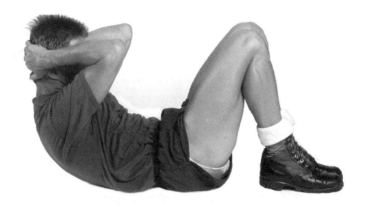

CRUNCHES — HEEL IN CLOSE

SEALs do Crunches with the heels in really close—as close as you can get them. Start with your hands behind your head as shown, knees bent and heels in tight, and using your abs, lift yourself to the crunch position. Do it slowly and with a controlled motion to get the most out of this crunch. Avoid pulling your head up with your hands! This is a sure way to strain your neck and cause injury.

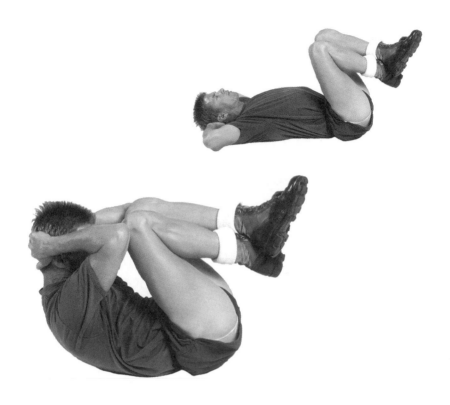

CRUNCHES — LEGS UP

The Legs Up Crunch is a traditional Navy SEAL ab exercise. A strong torso is a key to performing the many rigorous activities which are just a day's work for the SEALs. Doing Crunches will add to your overall ability to swim, run, climb ropes, and run the Obstacle Course, for example. Start with your hands behind your head as shown, legs up and knees bent at a 90° angle. Cross your ankles to create stability in your legs and lift yourself to the crunch position. Again, do it slowly and don't lift your head off the deck with your hands.

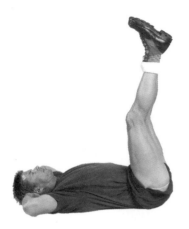

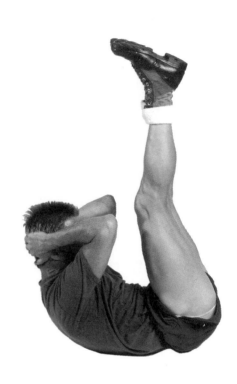

EXTENDED LEG CRUNCHES

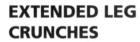

The Extended Leg Crunches are another variation. By extending your legs vertically, as shown, creating a 90° angle at the hips, you are able to concentrate all your firepower on your ab muscles. Keeping your legs in the air adds to the intensity of the crunch. Do these slowly and hold the crunch position for a two count if you desire a greater challenge.

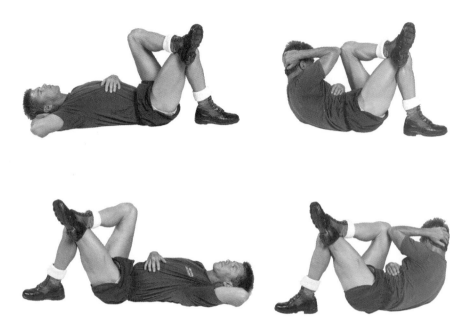

CROSS-LEGS SITUPS

This is designed as a Side Crunch for the intercostals, obliques, and serratus anterior. Start with your right leg up and flexed, your left leg crossed over it with your ankle on your knee. Then with your left hand on your abdomen and your right hand behind the head, move from the down position, flat on the deck, and lift your right elbow to meet your left knee. Do these slowly to maximize constant tension and peak contraction. Pause at the top, not at the bottom. And again, don't pull on your neck!

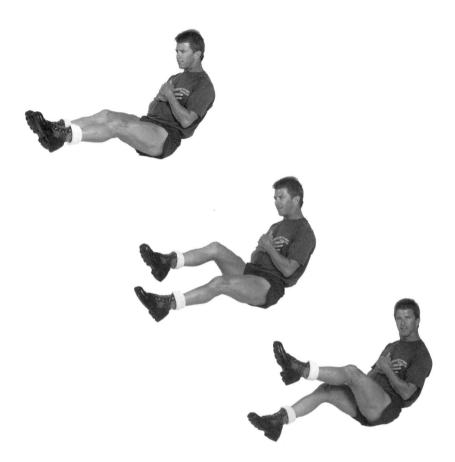

SITTING FLUTTER KICKS

With your butt on the deck, place your hands on your chest, legs up about six inches from the floor and start kicking. Keep your range of motion between six to 30 inches max. Again another fine way to prepare you for day-long ocean swims and underwater hydrographic reconnaissance missions.

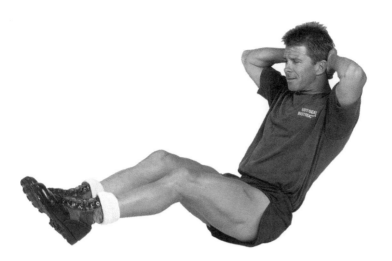

SITTING KNEE BENDERS

This is NOT an Atomic Situp! The major difference is that you start with your torso at a 45° angle to the ground. Extend your legs fully and keep your heels about six inches off the deck. Bring your knees in to meet your elbows. Extend your legs again. Repeat several times.

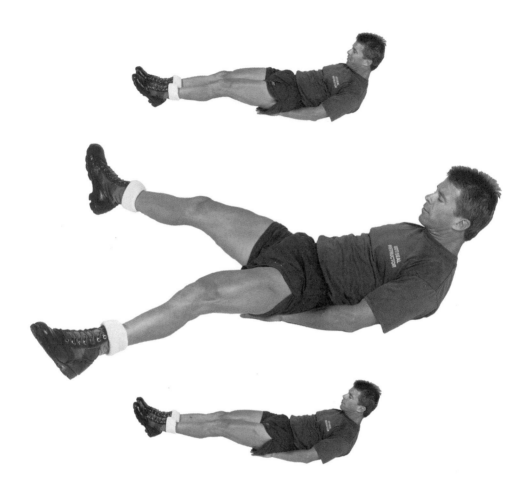

SCISSORS

Otherwise known as "Good Morning Darlings" at BUD/S, Scissors are another great way to strengthen your midsection. Lie on your back, cradling your torso with your arms as you did with the Leg Lever. Extend your legs out fully and keep your heels six inches off the deck. Open and close your legs as shown in the photo above. This exercise is counted in fours: open–close–open–close. One, two, three, ONE. One, two, three, TWO. One, two, three, THREE. Etc.

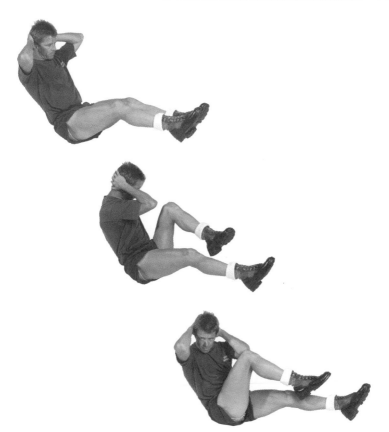

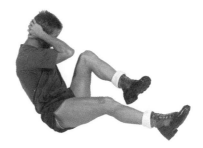

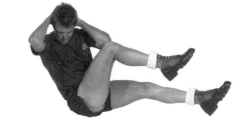

SITTING BICYCLES

The starting position is similar to the Sitting Knee Benders: hands behind head, torso at a 45° angle to the ground, legs fully extended, heels about six inches off the deck. Now, lift your knee as you twist your body and touch your knee with your opposite elbow. Think of your leg movement as if you were riding a bike. Alternate side-to-side in a continuous rhythmic motion.

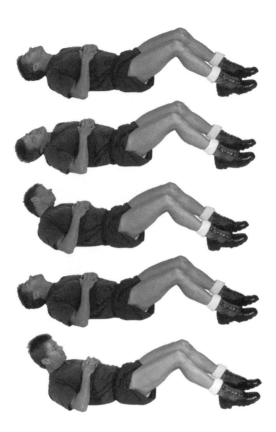

NECK ROTATIONS

It's not an ab exercise, but since you're on the deck now's as good time as any to do them. Strong neck muscles are important for one critical reason: to protect your neck and spine from sudden whip-type injuries. Think of the kind of things SEALs do and you will understand why: HALO parachuting from a C-130 transport, dropping 100 feet to the ocean from a Blackhawk helicopter, performing high-speed water insertions and retrievals. Any one of these can be potentially injurious if you have a weak neck. So don't forget to do these as part of your regular PT!

Keep it simple. Start on the deck. Legs comfortable as shown. Left-right-up-down. Reverse direction halfway through. Make that neck SEAL worthy! Hooyah!

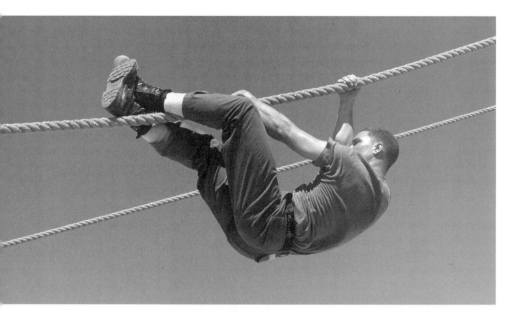

OBSTACLE
COURSE

The Obstacle Course is a major feature of SEAL training. It is another important component of the physical fitness readiness of each of the BUD/S students, and it builds confidence and competence physically.

A SEAL is made, not born. Watching SEALs fail, then gradually overcome the Obstacle Course is proof of this. There is a cross-section of people who enter SEAL training. There are great athletes. There are non-athletes, whose odds are against them but who make it nonetheless. In other words, a SEAL candidate is not necessarily a physical specimen. He could be someone with an average build, perhaps not uniquely successful as an athlete in high school, but somebody who has really got the grit and determination to stick with it.

The Obstacle Course is a measure of that spirit and determination that is an essential part of being a Navy SEAL. Are you ready? Then let's do it!

Parallel Bars → Low Wall → High Wall
↓

NAVY
SEAL
O'
COURSE

Vaulting Logs

↑

Spider Wall

↑

Incline Wall

↑

Tire Sequence

↑

Rope Swing

↑

Slide for Life Tower

↑

Barbed Wire

↓

Cargo Net

↓

Balance Logs

↓

Hooyah Logs

↓

Rope Transfer

↓

The Dirty Name

↓

More Hooyah Logs

← Burma Bridge ← The Weaver ←

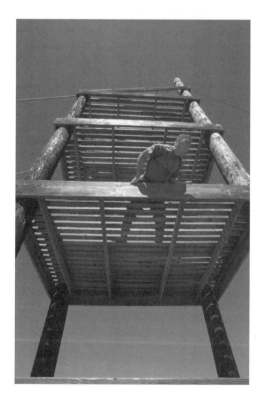

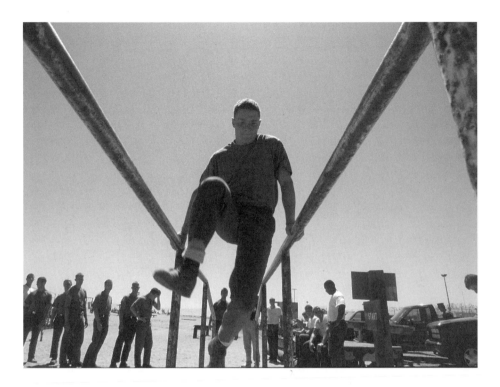

PARALLEL BARS

Traversing the Parallel Bars is like a moving Dip where you walk on your hands and bicycle pedal with your legs, or you can hop through on your hands. The length you must travel is about 20 feet. The bars are about five feet off the ground and they have an uphill section and then a flat section. You just work your way along. Easy day...so far. Then you run to the Low Wall.

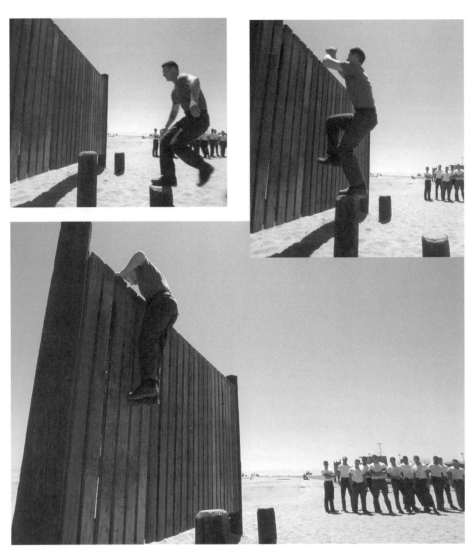

LOW WALL

The approach to the Low Wall is a series of telephone poles sawed down and stuck in the sand so they look like tree stumps. You leap from stump to stump and then launch yourself onto the Low Wall. It's only about 12 feet high. You jump onto it, grabbing the top with your hands, walking your feet up as you "mantle" or press up with your arms. Staying as low as you can and keeping your center of gravity down, you drop down on the other side.

Then there's a short run to the High Wall.

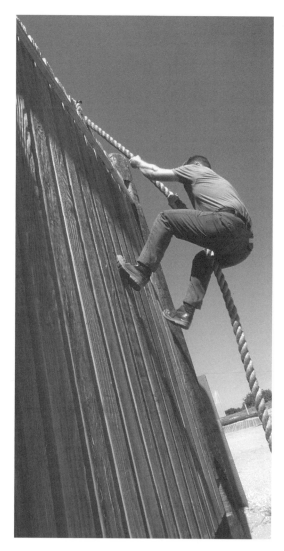

HIGH WALL

The face of the High Wall is sheathed with vertical boards. Suspended from the top of the Wall is an inviting and quite useful rope made of two-inch twisted manila hemp. Grabbing the rope, you climb up and hook a leg over the rail at the top, again keeping your center of gravity low, and swing over up onto the other side.

The key is to walk up the Wall, so you need to stay perpendicular to it. A lot of people tend to try to get upright—perpendicular to the ground—and that slows them down and their feet slide out from under them. But if you push away from it and just stay perpendicular to the Wall, you will succeed.

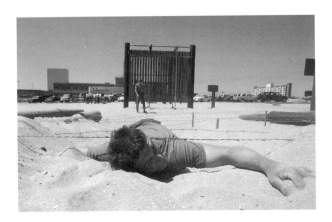

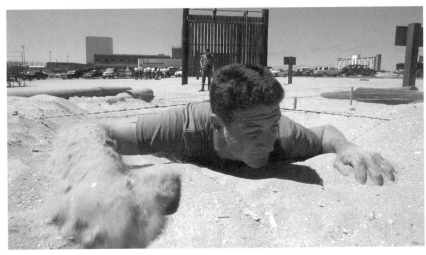

BARBED WIRE

Next you must crawl quickly underneath Barbed Wire. Barbed Wire is a feature of every traditional military obstacle course. The technique is to crawl on your belly, like a snake, and just pull yourself through, staying low and using your knees and elbows. You might take a little sand in your face here and there as you go through, but then again, this is SEAL training.

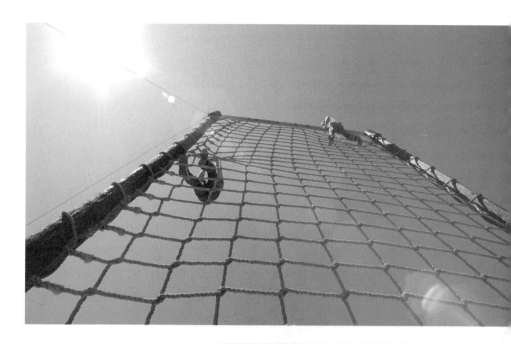

CARGO NET

Next you charge up the Cargo Net, over the rail, and down the other side. The Cargo Net rises to about 50 feet. The higher you go the more challenging it becomes. Although the Net is strung tightly and is replaced every six months, it still moves as you climb. The more SEALs on the Net, the more it moves and the more interesting it gets. SEALs learn to overcome their fear of heights quickly with the Cargo Net!

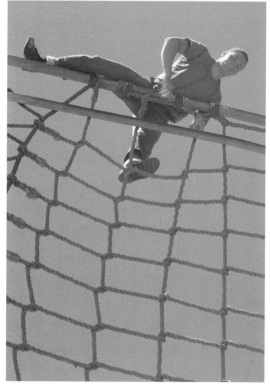

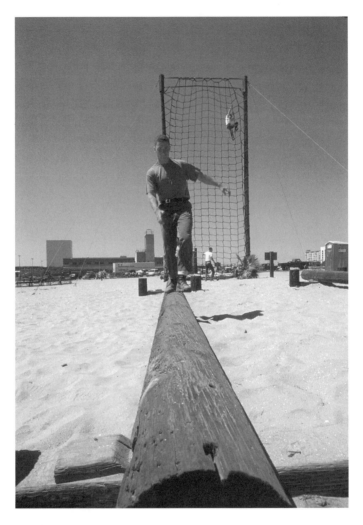

BALANCE LOGS

Next, there's a set of Balance Logs. There are three logs to negoti-
ate. You go down one, turn left, and then go straight again. The
logs are not fixed and they roll freely as you move along them, requiring you to keep your balance as you go.

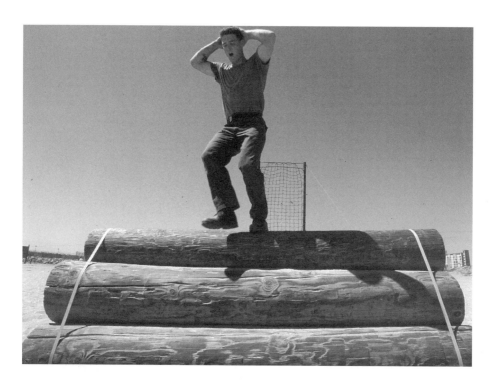

HOOYAH LOGS

The next obstacle is a set of ten logs stacked to form a pyramid. The SEALs call them Hooyah Logs because they run over them and say "Hooyah!" Although it's not required, many SEALs run them with their arms behind their heads...just for the challenge!

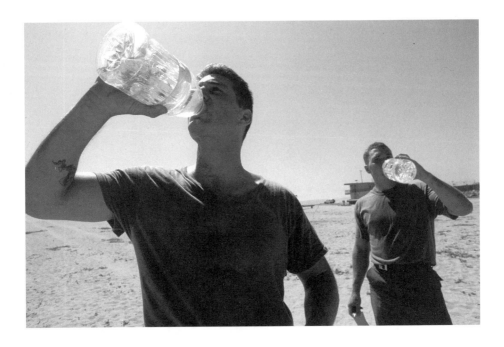

A WORD ON HYDRATION

Drinking plenty of water to stay hydrated is essential during workouts. Stop and drink water between sets of pushups and pull-ups and at any other logical breaks during your workout as well as before and after your workout—any time there is a break in the action.

Keep a supply of water handy. A used quart-sized sports drink bottle makes a great canteen.

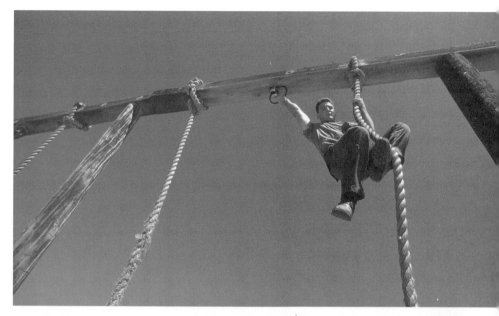

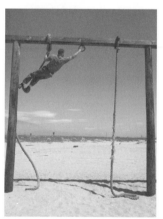 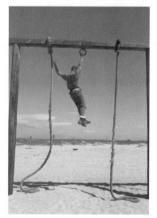 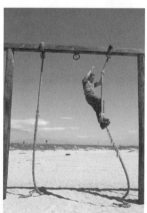

ROPE TRANSFER

Then there is the Rope Transfer. It's a real confidence and strength builder. The object is to climb up the rope to the left, grab the iron ring, then swing to the rope on the right and lower yourself down. On every obstacle proper technique is emphasized. When climbing and descending a rope, it is essential to maintain control to maximize speed and to minimize the risk of injury.

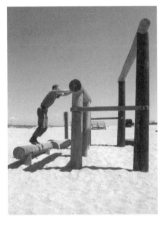 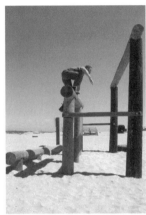 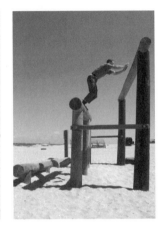

THE DIRTY NAME

When you see it, you know why it got its name! You vault off the bottom log, catching the middle log about hip level with your hands, and stand. If you think that's hard, you then have to launch yourself onto the higher log, catching it in the same manner with your hands at about hip level. Grabbing the high log you swing up and roll yourself over the top. Drop to the ground and you are done with the Dirty Name. At least for today.

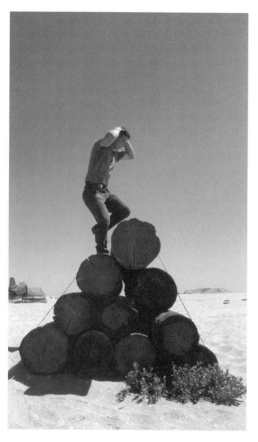 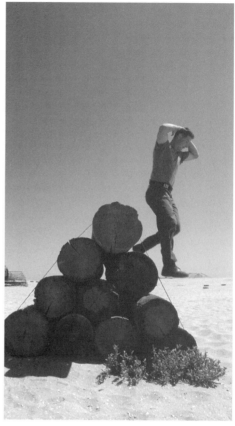

MORE HOOYAH LOGS

Then there are more Hooyah Logs to run over. Everyone likes the Hooyah Logs. It gives you a few moments to rest and recover some upper body strength before the next obstacle: the Weaver.

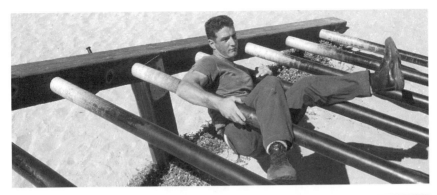

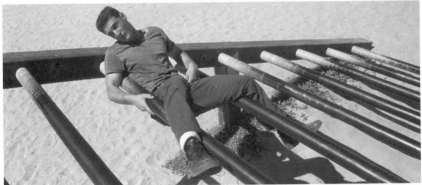

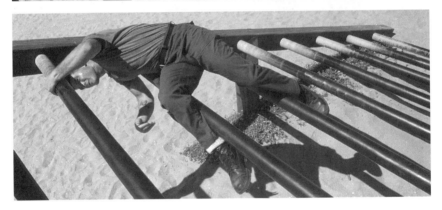

THE WEAVER

The Weaver is a really strange looking obstacle. It is a pyramid-shaped structure rising to about six feet. Built mostly of parallel iron pipes, it requires you to travel under one pipe and over the next, up to the high point and down the other side, weaving your way through it. Negotiating the Weaver takes a lot of coordination. SEALs find it's highly effective in slowing down overall completion times on the obstacle course...not that you needed help with that!

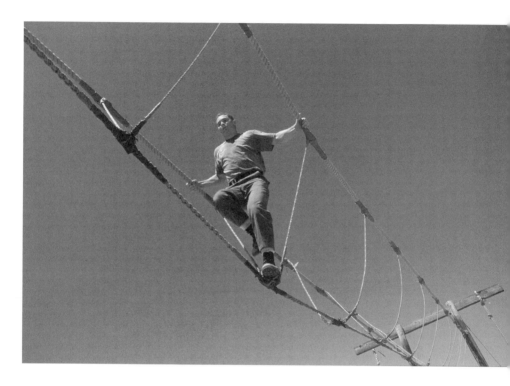

BURMA BRIDGE

Another classic military obstacle. The bridge extends about 75 feet in length and is accessed by a rope climb of about 12 feet. Traversing the Burma Bridge requires balance and coordination. The rope tends to pitch and sway as you go, the hand rails providing only a minimum of assistance. Descent from the Burma Bridge is also by rope.

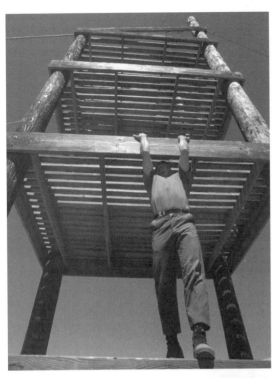

SLIDE FOR LIFE TOWER

The Slide for Life Tower is perhaps the most awesome and intimidating obstacle on the course. Here's a four-story tower (about 40 feet) that you first must ascend without the aid of ladders or steps, then you must descend from the top on one of two 100-foot ropes leading to the ground at a gentle angle.

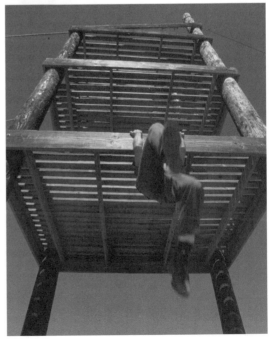

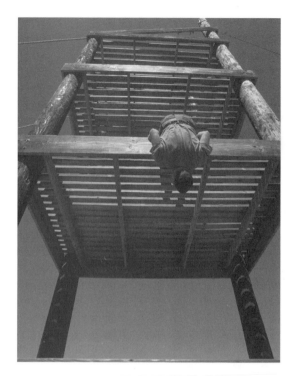

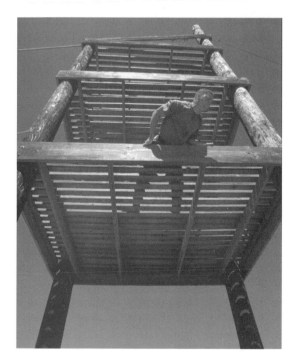

To climb up the tower, most SEALs use one of two techniques: the leg-over or the back flip. The leg-over is performed by first pulling yourself up by your arms (much like a pull-up) then throwing a leg over the top. You can use your heel to hook over the edge and then pull your body onto the next platform. It's certainly not a graceful technique but it gets the job done.

The back-flip method is just that. Facing outward, you grab the platform above you curl-up style and then using your momentum you flip yourself back over onto the next level. It is definitely the most efficient way to climb the Tower once perfected, but until then...practice at lower levels!

95

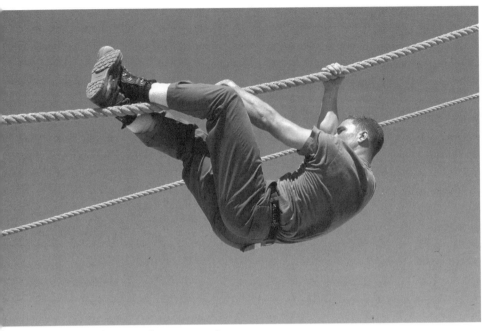

Rope descent banana style

Descent from the Tower on the Slide for Life is performed in one of two ways. You can descend "Banana Style," used during First and Second Phase of BUD/S, or you can descend "Commando Style" once you have entered Third Phase. Lowering yourself Banana Style is tough on the arms and legs. You are upside down and pulling yourself along hand over hand, with gravity working against you all the way down. Once you have mastered the Commando Style descent, it's much easier. Commando Style demands more agility and balance, but it is by far less exhausting. By Third Phase, SEAL candidates have had a lot of opportunity to hone their balance skills.

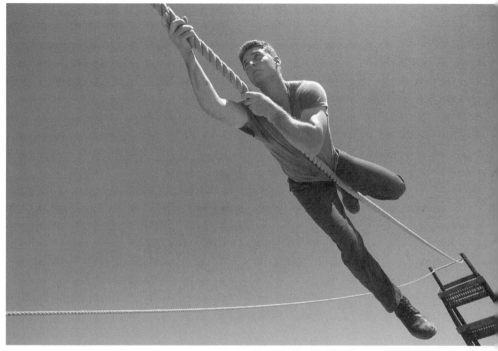

Commando style

SAFETY IS A #1 CONCERN

The Slide for Life Tower presents an excellent opportunity to mention safety. Many people ask, "Do people ever fall off the Tower?" Safety is a primary concern of the Navy SEALs, and especially of the instructors at BUD/S. A SEAL's job is dangerous enough, so why take unneeded risks? At the BUD/S Obstacle Course there is always a corpsman present as well as a safety officer. There is emergency transportation available, too. If for some reason a safety officer is not present, the Cargo Net and the Slide for Life Tower are omitted from the course that day.

If on the Slide for Life Tower a SEAL candidate thinks he is going to fall, he has been instructed to drop his legs, hang on with his hands, then fall feet first. It's soft sand and this controlled falling technique usually prevents injury. Still, some students fall without control, and the corpsman is prepared to provide aid if they do injure themselves.

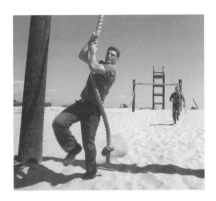

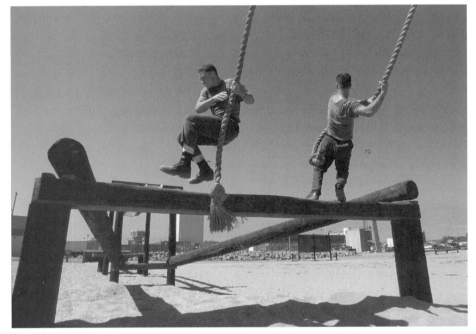

ROPE SWING

Once you have lowered yourself from the Slide for Life Tower, you proceed to the Rope Swing. The Rope Swing is harder than it looks. Using a rope, you swing from the sand to a log about four feet off the ground. You must land firmly on this log and let go of the rope quickly, or else you will find yourself eating sand. It's another example of proper technique winning over brute strength.

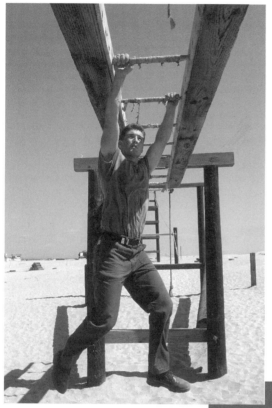

It's a quick walk down fixed logs to the Monkey Bars, which you travel hand over hand—just like when you were a kid. Only now you are in the hot sun and some other guy is coming up right behind you fast and it feels as if you've been doing this kind thing all day—because you have. Finishing the Monkey Bars you run along another fixed log (it's getting easier) and it's a quick sprint through the Tires.

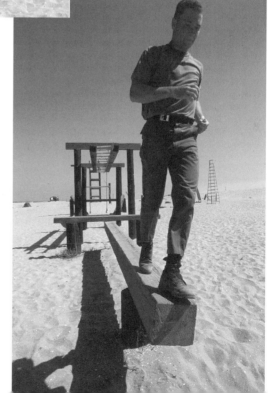

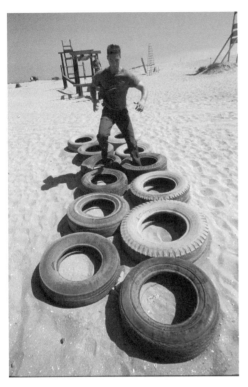

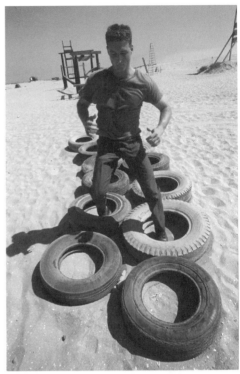

TIRE SEQUENCE

Hit the holes and not the rims as you make a dash for the Incline Wall.

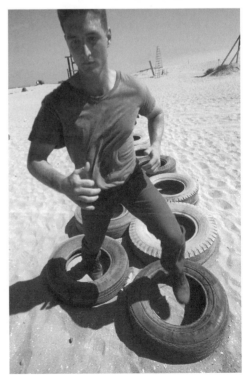

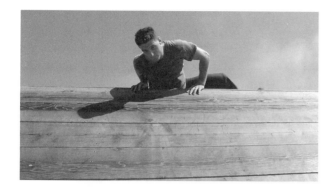

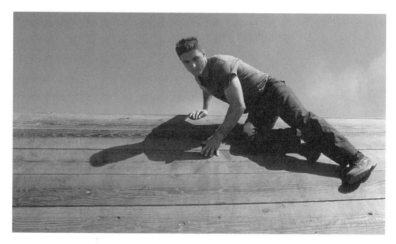

INCLINE WALL

Hop up and slide (or run down) the face. Piece of cake. Easy day. Wouldn't it be nice if all obstacles would be so gentle? Not so: Soon we will be burning our forearms on the Spider Wall.

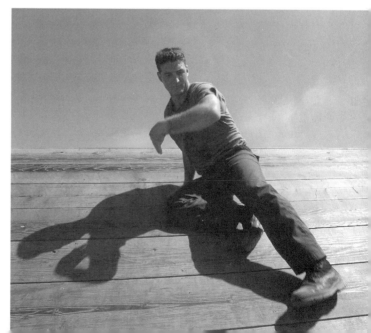

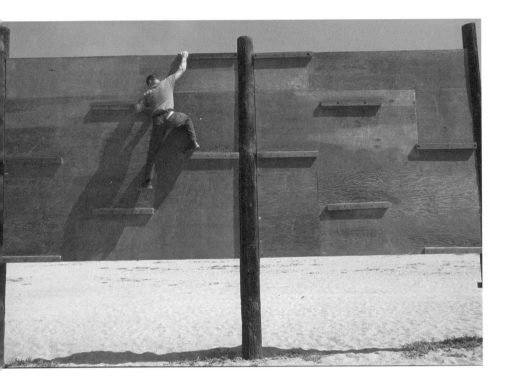

SPIDER WALL

The Spider Wall is quite similar to a climbing wall, and teaches similar skills. Balance, technique, agility—all come into play on the Spider Wall. The key is to use your legs to push yourself up rather than your arms. If you were to rely mostly on your arms on the Spider Wall your forearms would burn out before you completed the required traverse of the obstacle. Trust your legs and use your arms and hands as little as possible except for balance. You will feel great when you discover how easy it can be using proper climbing technique. We're almost done!

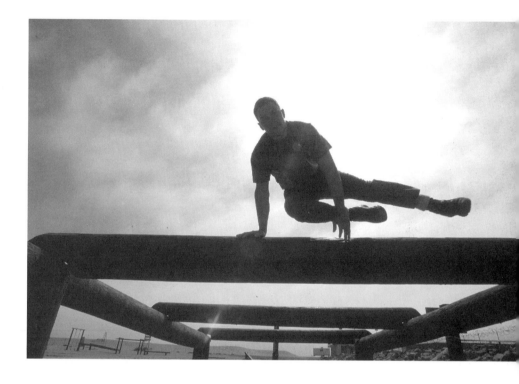

VAULTING LOGS

The last obstacle is the Vaulting Logs. They are a series of evenly spaced telephone poles parallel to the ground and about four feet high. The only rule: no touching with your legs or feet. You must hurdle over the logs quickly because time is running out.

Charge to the end. Give the BUD/S instructor and your classmates 20 perfect pushups. Stand up and say:

"Hooyah O'Course"

You're done! Easy day.

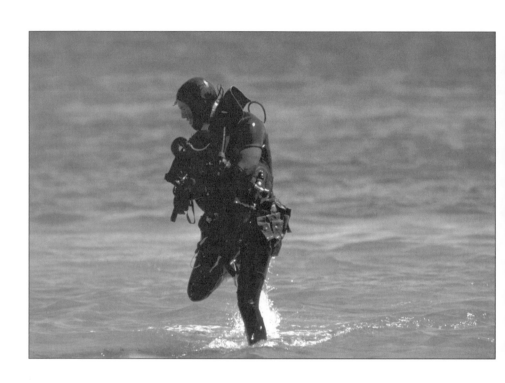

NAVY SEAL NUTRITION

You can't achieve peak fitness without paying attention to what you eat. Strong dietary habits are critical both before entering BUD/S training and during the training itself. Optimum performance is achieved by proper nutrient intake and is essential to receiving maximum performance output during exercise. Nutrition also promotes vital muscle and tissue growth and repair. The ideal diet provides all the nutrients that the body needs and supplies energy for exercise.

Balancing energy intake and expenditure can be very difficult when activity levels are very high (as in SEAL training) and when activity levels are very low, such as during isolation. Typically, body weight remains constant when energy intake equals expenditure.

You can upset this "energy balance equation" by increasing or decreasing the number of calories you consume, increasing or decreasing your energy expenditure, or both. One pound of body fat is equal to 3500 calories. So to lose 1 pound in 1 week, you'd have to, over the course of the week, consume 3500 fewer calories, increase your activity level, or a combination of the two. To gain 1 pound in the same time, you'd need to consume 3500 calories more than you expend, decrease your physical activity, or a combination of both.

COMPONENTS OF ENERGY EXPENDITURE

The three major contributors to energy expenditure are:
- Resting energy expenditure (REE)
- Physical activity
- Energy used to digest foods.

The first two contributors are most pertinent to our discussion. Resting energy expenditure (REE) is the amount of energy required to maintain life—your breathing, heartbeat, body temperature regulation, and other life processes (but not physical exertion). You can estimate your REE with the following formula.

Determining Resting Energy Expenditure (REE) of Men from Body Weight (in Pounds)

Age (years)	Equation to Derive REE (cal/day)
18 to 30	6.95 x Weight + 679
30 to 60	5.27 x Weight + 879

To calculate your total daily caloric expenditure you need to account for your physical activity in addition to your REE. The amount of energy SEAL trainees expend during training varies from day to day. Some days are very strenuous and involve running, swimming, calisthenics, cold water exposure, sleep deprivation, and carrying heavy loads. Some days are spent in the classroom sitting a good portion of the time. Thus, determining your actual energy expended during activity is more difficult. But there are ways to estimate. One is to multiply your REE by an "activity factor."

Estimating Total Daily Energy Needs of Men at Various Levels of Activity

Level of Activity	Activity Factor
Very Light (Seated and standing activities, driving, playing cards)	1.3
Light (Walking, carpentry, sailing, ping-pong, pool, or golf)	1.6
Moderate (Carrying a load, jogging, light swimming, biking, calisthenics, scuba diving)	1.7
Heavy (Walking with a load uphill, rowing, digging, climbing, soccer, basketball, running, obstacle course)	2.1

Level of Activity	Activity Factor
Exceptional (Running/swimming races, biking uphill, carrying very heavy loads, hard rowing)	2.4

Here's an example using a 21-year-old male who weighs 175 pounds and whose activity level is moderate:

REE = 6.95 x 175[1] + 679 = 1895 calories per day

Total Energy Needs = 1895 x 1.7[2] = **3222 calories per day**

[1] weight in pounds [2] "Moderate" Activity Factor

Body Mass Index

The Body Mass Index (BMI) is a measure commonly used to assess body composition and then classify individuals as underweight, overweight, or overfat. The BMI is a ratio: weight/height^2, with weight measured in kilograms and height in meters.

The reference ranges developed for the United States population (see page 108) as a whole do not always apply to special populations such as the SEALs. For that reason, a BMI reference range based on a survey of 800 SEALs was developed. For all SEALs combined, the average BMI was 25 and the average body fat was 13 percent. What is important to remember is that the index is a screening tool. You can use the BMI to assess and keep track of changes in your body composition. If your BMI is high, have your body fat checked. If it's more than 20 percent, you need to take some action to lower your weight. Reference BMI values for you are provided below:

Reference BMI Values for SEALs

Lean	<20
Typical SEAL	**20 to 29**
Overfat	29 to 32

EATING FOR OPTIMUM HEALTH

Once you know where you stand in terms of your BMI, caloric intake, and caloric expenditures, it's important to carefully consider your diet. The following section is dedicated to explaining the way to build a healthful diet that will see you through SEAL training. The information

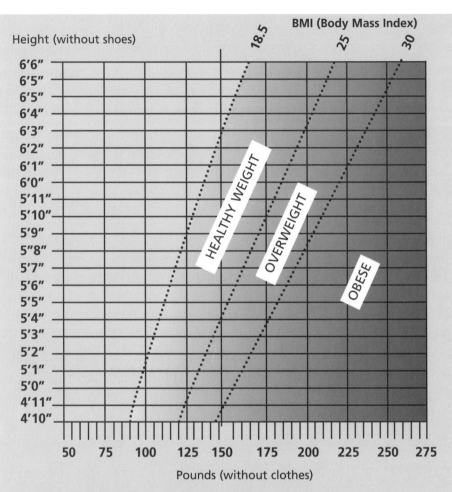

Pounds (without clothes)

BMI measures weight in relation to height. The BMI ranges shown above are for adults. They are not exact ranges of healthy and unhealthy weights. However, they show that health risk increases at higher levels of overweight and obesity. Even within the healthy BMI range, weight gains can carry health risks for adults.

Directions: Find your weight on the bottom of the graph. Go straight up from that point until you come to the line that matches your height. Then look to find your weight group.

Healthy Weight: BMI from 18.5 up to 25 refers to a healthy weight.

Overweight: BMI from 25 up to 30 refers to overweight.

Obese: BMI 30 or higher refers to obesity. Obese persons are also overweight.

comes from the Dietary Guidelines for Americans released in 2000 by the U.S. Department of Agriculture and the U.S. Department of Health and Human Services. Top dietitians and scientists have studied the practicality and reliability of the data. It is tested, supported, credentialed. It works.

In this section you'll learn about basic nutrition: Your daily nutrient needs. Your daily caloric needs. Vitamins, minerals, and more. From there you'll discover the Food Pyramid. It's a simple yet profound way to understand where your calories should come from. Finally, you'll learn how to read a nutrition label and be able to make intelligent, healthy decisions at the supermarket or even at a fast food restaurant.

THE CHALLENGE OF CHOICE

Good nutrition boils down to two elements: choice and portion size. Choice involves the types of foods you eat and how they're prepared. Are you more apt to eat a baked sweet potato or plate of fries? An apple or apple pie? Even the simplest choices, such as the decision to forego slabs of butter on your pancakes, can save you hundreds of calories that you probably won't even miss in terms of flavor.

As important as *what* you eat is *how much* of each food you eat. There are no good or bad foods (with the exception of trans-fatty acids, which are covered later). Portion control is the key. In the last few years portion sizes of virtually all foods—from mega-muffins, to "big grab" chips to cookies to restaurant entreés—have ballooned. Often, what is sold in single packages really represents two or three servings. In this section you'll also find out how to determine sensible portion sizes based on the Pyramid model.

The Food Guide Pyramid

Fad diets come and go, but basic science-backed nutrition advice has remained remarkably consistent. In fact, many reported studies have proven that the best way to lose fat, keep it off, and to enjoy a healthful diet is to follow a plan that is rooted not in a new trend, but in the Department of Agriculture's Food Guide Pyramid. While most of us are excited by new trends and fads, the truth is that they don't work in the long term. What does work is a balanced eating and exercising plan that is based on reasonable and attainable goals.

The key to the Food Guide Pyramid is that it provides a wide range of

Popular Diets Analyzed

Here's a critical look at some of today's most popular diet programs.

Low-Carbohydrate, High-Protein Initially these diets seem to work. Weight loss is quick the first week or two, but the loss is primarily water. When your body has exhausted its carbohydrate supply, it manufactures sugar from protein, including muscle protein. Your muscle tissue burns calories like crazy; fat is hardly burned at all. The large amount of muscle loss means caloric needs decrease significantly; weight loss stops, and frustration sets in. When a normal diet is resumed, the pounds return. In many instances, you end up heavier than when you started, because your metabolic rate decreases along with your muscle loss.

Many low-carbohydrate, high-protein diet books ignore recommendations from the American Heart, Dietetic, and Diabetes associations as well as those of the USDA. These authorities develop guidelines for optimal health based on extensive scientific research.

Low-carbohydrate, high-protein diets, over the short term, can cause constipation, dizziness, irritability, bad breath, improper kidney functioning, a loss of sodium and dehydration. Long-term effects may increase the risk for developing heart attacks, strokes and cancer.

Formula Diets So-called formula diets—those in which low-calorie liquids are consumed—have been around for years. Most of these provide adequate nutrition with the exception of dietary fiber. But boredom can set in quickly and the formula loses its appeal. Since reasonable eating habits were not learned while consuming these low-calorie drinks, the weight is rapidly regained when the formula is abandoned.

High-Fiber Diets High-fiber diets are based on several theories: Fiber, when combined with water, causes bulk in the intestines and creates a feeling of fullness. Because most fiber-rich foods take a long time to chew, you don't have time to overeat. The result? Fewer calories are consumed. Generally, high-fiber foods are low in calories and high in nutrition. Thus, most high-fiber diets are nutritionally sound. Just be sure you also eat adequate amounts of other foods. Let the Food Pyramid be your guide. Note: Don't increase your fiber too rapidly or constipation will set in, and make sure your water consumption rises simultaneously for the same reason.

choices so you can eat a variety of tasty foods. Eating a variety of foods ensures that you get all the important nutrients, vitamins, and minerals that your body requires for optimal health. It also means that you won't be bored to death because you can select different foods every day.

The Food Guide Pyramid provides shows the types and quantities of foods you should eat every day. It's broken into six food groups: grains, vegetables, fruits, dairy, proteins, and fats and sweets. Most of your diet should come from the foods at the base of the Pyramid (the grains group); the least amount should come from those at the top (fats, oils and sweets). You'll notice that you can have six to 11 servings of grains each day, which are rich in carbohydrates.

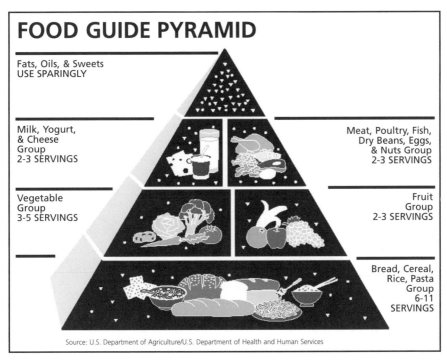

FOOD GUIDE PYRAMID

Fats, Oils, & Sweets
USE SPARINGLY

Milk, Yogurt,
& Cheese
Group
2-3 SERVINGS

Meat, Poultry, Fish,
Dry Beans, Eggs,
& Nuts Group
2-3 SERVINGS

Vegetable
Group
3-5 SERVINGS

Fruit
Group
2-3 SERVINGS

Bread, Cereal,
Rice, Pasta
Group
6-11
SERVINGS

Source: U.S. Department of Agriculture/U.S. Department of Health and Human Services

The Importance of Fruits and Vegetables

In addition to choosing healthy grains, try to eat at least five servings of fruits and vegetables every day. This is essential. Many scientific studies have shown that people whose diets are plentiful in fruits and vegetables have reduced risk for many diseases, including a variety of cancers. Fruits and vegetables are great sources of essential vitamins, minerals, and fiber. Unfortunately, most of us do not eat the five recommended servings daily; and if we do, we eat the less healthy vegetables, such as iceberg lettuce, rather than the nutrient-dense dark greens. Dark green leafy vegetables, deeply colored fruits, and beans and peas are very rich in vitamins and minerals. A good rule of thumb is to make your plate as colorful as possible with a variety of vegetables to be sure you are getting all the nutrients you need.

How can you make sure you eat enough from this food group? Choose chopped vegetables as a snack when you feel hungry; or grab an apple instead of a candy bar. Drink juice instead of soda. Prepare salads with tomatoes, cucumbers, peppers, and other vegetables. Soon you'll see how easy it really is to eat those five servings.

DAILY NUTRIENT NEEDS

For a healthy, balanced diet, you need to consume healthful portions of protein, carbohydrates, fats, vitamins and minerals, and water. Here's the breakdown. Keep in mind that the following recommended daily amounts are for normal, healthy adults of average size.

Protein
Protein is made up of chemicals called amino acids. Some types of amino acids—called *nonessential amino acids*—are are produced by the body. Nine *essential amino acids* must come from food you consume. Protein allows the body to build, maintain, and replace body tissue. Muscles, organs, and some hormones are made up primarily of protein. Protein also makes hemoglobin, the part of red blood cells that carries oxygen, and antibodies, the cells that fight off infection and disease.

Beans, cheese, chicken, eggs, fish, meat, and nuts are all good sources of protein. The recommended daily intake of protein is 50 to 70 grams (which should equal 12 to 20 percent of your daily caloric intake).

Carbohydrates
There are two types of carbohydrates: simple and complex. Simple carbohydrates are sugars. They're quickly and easily broken down and digested by the body. Complex carbohydrates, also known as starches, take longer to be digested than simple carbohydrates.

Carbohydrates are the preferred energy source for physical activity. It takes at least 20 hours after demanding exercise to restore muscle energy, provided 600 grams of carbohydrates are consumed each day. During successive days of exhausting training like that at BUD/S, your energy stores become depleted. A high-carbohydrate diet can help you maintain energy.

Good sources of simple carbohydrates include fruits, such as apples,

Naval Special Warfare Center Dietary Supplement Policy

1. Individually packaged (single-serving) Gatorade or PowerAde electrolyte (salt) replacement drinks are allowed.

2. Only vitamins dispensed by Naval Special Warfare Center (NSWC) Medical will be used if you desire a multi-vitamin supplement.

3. Protein powder, although discouraged, may be used. The product must be in single-serving packets, (i.e. myoplex envelopes) and must be cleared and stamped by NSWC Medical prior to use and storage within barracks, automobiles, etc.

4. Glucosamine and Chondroitin Sulfate will be prescribed by NSWC Medical Officers for staff/students/trainees with extensive (documented) joint and cartilage disorders on a case-by-case basis.

Prohibited Supplements at NSWC and BUD/S All other supplements are strictly prohibited. This includes all herbal and non-herbal supplements in addition to: Anabolic steroids, creatine, ephedrine/ephedra containing compounds, metabolic boosters, Ma Huang, Guarana, DHEA, and the like.

Allowed Dietary Supplements at NSWC and BUD/S In general, the NSWC student/trainee will learn proper nutrition by focusing on quality foods with high nutritional value (i.e. boiled eggs, tuna fish, lean meats, fresh fruits and vegetables, peanut butter, breads and cereals, cheese, yogurts and other dairy products, milk, and the like). Navy chow halls/messing facilities provide more than adequate macronutrients for the demands of BUD/S, SWCC, SQT and other NSWC courses.

All NSWC students/trainees are allowed double quantity food rations during scheduled chow hall hours—just politely ask your server to double your rations. Train smarter, not poorer—do not fall prey to the dietary and sports nutrition industry. Your UDT/Frogman and Special Boat Service forefathers did not need supplements and neither do you!

bananas, grapes, raisins, oranges, and pears. Good sources of complex carbohydrates include bread, cereals, pasta, rice, oatmeal, pretzels, corn, potatoes, sweet potatoes, tomatoes, carrots, cucumbers, lettuce, and peppers.

For most healthy individuals, the recommended intake of carbohydrates is 350 to 400 grams per day or 55 to 65 percent of your daily caloric intake. During the rigors of SEAL training, however, about 600 grams per day or up to 70 percent of your daily caloric intake should be from carbohydrates. Most of that should come from foods that are high in complex carbohydrates.

Fat

You may have noticed that the Pyramid Guide allows you to consume 25 to 30 percent of your daily calories from fat. For too long Americans have bought into the myth that fat is evil and that severely controlling fat intake would control weight. This was based largely on the fact that high-fat foods contain more calories per gram than do other foods. (A single gram of fat has 9 calories; a single gram of carbohydrates and protein has 4 calories.) However, substituting non-fat or low-fat products for fats has not led to success in fat loss. Why? Here are the facts about fat.

FACT: Fat-free does not equal calorie-free. Many no-fat or low-fat foods are high in sugar, which often significantly increases their calorie content. In addition, people tend to eat larger portions of fat-free foods, thereby increasing the amount of calories consumed.

FACT: Fat satiates. In general, you need to eat less of a food with fat than you do of a non-fat food to feel full. For this reason, many people tend to overeat non-fat or low-fat foods.

FACT: You *need* some fat. This one is hard for people to accept, but it is true. Fat is a major nutrient that is vital for proper growth and development and maintenance of good health. Certain vitamins (A, E, and K) are soluble only in fat.

However, not all fats are healthful. In general, you should steer clear of saturated fats, which are artery cloggers. You'll find them in butter, meats, and palm and coconut oils. Also avoid trans-fatty acids (fats that are formed when foods are hydrogenated and that are found in deep-fried commercial foods and many packaged foods, especially baked goods). These fats act like saturated fats but are even worse: In addition to raising levels of so-called "bad" cholesterol (known as LDL) in our bodies (as saturated fats do), they lower the levels of the "good" cholesterol (HDL), which are necessary to keep our arteries clear.

Monosaturated and polyunsaturated fats are the "good" fats. They're found in foods including olive oil and canola oil and are absolutely necessary for many functions of life. Our bodies also require essential fatty acids (EFAs), such as linoleic and alpha linoleic acid, for normal cell growth and development. The only way to get these fatty acids is through your diet. EFAs are found primarily in fatty fish, such as salmon and mackerel, and in certain nuts, oils, and dark green vegetables. There is significant evidence that a diet rich in essential fatty acids can protect against heart disease. Recently, the American Heart Association, recognizing the important heart protective role that these fatty acids play, revised its dietary guidelines to include suggesting that we eat two servings of fatty fish each week.

Recommended daily intake of fat is 30 to 65 grams per day (approximately 25 to 30 percent of your caloric intake).

Vitamins and Minerals

When it comes to supplementing our diets with vitamins people can be passionate. Some people strongly believe that taking vitamin supplements each day is necessary to maintain or improve their health. But vitamins are not subject to Food and Drug Administration (FDA) approval, and so manufacturers have wide leeway in marketing these products. Be careful about taking any vitamins in very large doses (100 times the RDA), because they can be toxic at these levels.

Vitamins and minerals are found in the foods we eat and most nutrition experts agree that the best way to get vitamins is by consuming a healthy diet. So, if you eat a healthy diet based on the Pyramid guidelines you probably will get all the vitamins and minerals you need. However, many of us because of poor eating habits, have developed deficiencies—most commonly in folate, vitamin B6, antioxidants, calcium, and zinc. Taking a daily multivitamin—one that does not exceed the recommended nutrient levels—may be a good way to insure that you receive adequate amounts of these nutrients.

Antioxidants are important compounds that preserve and protect your body's cells from the damage of free radicals. Free radicals are oxygen molecules that have split into single electron molecules and that can cause tissue damage. Beta carotene, vitamins C and E, and the minerals sulfur and selenium are powerful antioxidants. The following checklists provide the US RDA for the major vitamins and minerals for adults and children over four. Bear in mind that your age and certain health conditions may call for you to have more or less of a particular vitamin or mineral. Check with your doctor.

Water

Water, which comprises about 75 percent of our total body weight, serves many functions. It helps regulate our body temperature: When we sweat, we rid ourselves of excess heat. Water transports needed nutrients to our cells and removes toxic substances and wastes. It cushions our body tissues and lubricates our joints. Water provides moisture for our respiratory system and is essential for our digestion. Since water is a major component of all cell structures, including muscle structure and function, it takes second place only to oxygen as the most important body component. Unfortunately, most people often overlook this fact.

Since our bodies cannot store or conserve water, it is critical to drink adequate amounts of it every day, especially in hot weather and during physical training. In general, you should consume up to four quarts a day (that's 12 to 16 eight-ounce glasses). Ideally you should drink water in intervals throughout the day. Keep a bottle with you at all times so that you can easily take regular drinks. When you exercise you should drink one to two cups of water an hour before you begin and then an additional four to eight ounces every 15 minutes during your workout.

Substances such as alcohol, caffeine, and tobacco increase your body's need for water. Consumed in excess, these substances will harm your body and hinder your performance. Not drinking enough water during physical training or on hot days can result in lack of coordination, irritability, fatigue, muscle cramping, mental confusion—and even more severe problems. Water intake is vital, so stay hydrated!

READING FOOD LABELS

Learning how to interpret the information on food labels gives you a valuable nutrition tool. First, look at the front panel of a food, which lists any nutrients that have been added. For example, a cereal with "fortified" or "enriched" on the front panel may mean that certain vitamins and/or minerals have been added to the grain. Furthermore, the ingredients listed first are the ones present in the highest concentrations by weight. Too often those ingredients are sugar and sodium. Shop for foods that have healthy ingredients front and center.

The serving sizes listed on labels can also be misleading, so you need to examine them carefully. For instance, the label on a small bag of potato chips may list "150 calories per serving," which doesn't sound like much. But read the label more carefully, and you may find that the bag contains three servings, not just one. If you eat all of the chips in the bag, you'll have consumed 450 calories.

Finally, it is helpful to know how to convert the nutrients presented

What Counts as a Serving?

The Food Guide Pyramid tells us to eat a particular number of servings per day of each kind of food: 3 servings of meat, 3 servings of milk, and so forth. But what exactly is one serving?

Milk, Yogurt, and Cheese
Eat 2 to 3 servings every day
1 serving equals 1 1/2 ounces of natural cheese OR 2 ounces of process cheese OR 8 ounces of yogurt OR 8 ounces of milk.

Meat, Poultry, Fish
Eat 2 to 3 servings every day
1 serving equals 2 to 3 ounces of cooked lean meat, poultry, or fish. 1/2 cup of cooked dry beans OR 1 egg OR 2 tablespoons peanut butter count as 1 ounce of lean meat.

Vegetables
Eat 3 to 5 servings every day
1 serving equals 1 cup of raw leafy vegetables OR 1/2 cup of other vegetables, cooked or chopped raw OR 3/4 cup of vegetable juice.

Fruit
Eat 2 to 4 servings every day
1 serving equals 1 medium apple, banana, or orange OR 1/2 cup of chopped, cooked, or canned fruit OR 3/4 cup of fruit juice.

Cereal, Rice, and Pasta
Eat 6 to 11 servings every day
1 serving equals 1 slice of bread OR 1 ounce of ready-to-eat cereal OR 1/2 cup of cooked cereal, rice, or pasta.

on the label in grams to calories to determine how much (energy-wise) of each individual nutrient you would be eating in a serving.

Carbohydrates	1 gram equals 4 calories
Proteins	1 gram equals 4 calories
Fats	1 gram equals 9 calories

When reading a label pay attention to the amount of cholesterol and sodium; many low-fat and low-calorie foods are high in sodium (healthy adults should consume no more than 2400 mg per day.) And check to see whether the food contains saturated or hydrogenated oils;

if it does, you may want to avoid it, because hydrogenated foods contain trans-fatty acids (see page 114).

Here are some more label reading tips:

- Note the order of ingredients listed (those most abundant appear first).
- Read the nutrient information to determine the relative amounts of protein, carbs, fats, vitamins, and minerals the food provides.
- Check the serving size: Beware! Many packages contain two or three servings.
- Avoid foods that contain hydrogenated oils.
- Look for foods that strike a Pyramid-based balance among carbohydrates, fats, and proteins.

On the following pages you'll find Vitamin and Mineral Checklists. Each contains information about the function of each nutrient and each lists those foods that contain the highest concentrations of each vitamin and mineral. Eat the foods recommended on these checklists and you can be confident that you're giving your body the right nutrients you need for good health—and for the rigorous demands of physical training like that of BUD/S training.

VITAMIN CHECKLIST

VITAMIN A
Functions
> prevents night blindness, keeps body tissues healthy, allows for normal bone and teeth growth

Best Food Sources
> dark, green leafy vegetables, red, orange, or yellow vegetables and fruits, liver, eggs, fish oils, and fortified foods such as milk

Requirements
> 800 to 1000 microgram retinol equivalents

Deficiency
> poor night vision, increased risk of osteomalacia (soft bones), and osteoporosis

Toxicity
> liver damage, bone abnormalities, headaches, double vision, hair loss, vomiting

118

VITAMIN D
Functions
promotes strong bones and teeth
Best Food Sources
eggs, cheese, sardines, fortified milk, cereals, and margarine
Requirements
5 to 10 micrograms
Deficiency
increased osteoporosis and osteomalacia risk
Toxicity
weak muscles and bones, kidney stones and damage, excessive bleeding

VITAMIN E
Functions
helps form cell membranes, increases resistance to disease and possibly reduces the risk of certain cancers as well as heart disease
Best Food Sources
vegetable oils, seeds, nuts, and wheat germ
Requirements
8 to 10 mg alpha-tocopherol equivalents
Deficiency
abnormal nervous system functioning, premature, very low birth weight infants
Toxicity
unknown, but very high amounts may interfere with the functioning of other nutrients

VITAMIN K
Functions
promotes normal blood clotting
Best Food Sources
green leafy vegetables
Requirements
55 to 80 micrograms
Deficiency
abnormal blood clotting
Toxicity
none known

VITAMIN C

Functions
repairs damaged tissues, promotes wound healing, increases resistance to infection, maintains healthy gums, bones, and teeth

Best Food Sources
citrus fruits and juices, strawberries, tomatoes, potatoes, and raw cabbage

Requirements
60 milligrams

Deficiency
scurvy (symptoms may include bleeding, improper wound healing, loose teeth, and swollen gums)

Toxicity
gastrointestinal pain and diarrhea

VITAMIN B1 (THIAMIN)

Functions
carbohydrate metabolism

Best Food Sources
whole grains, nuts, peas, beans, pork, enriched breads and cereals

Requirements
1 to 1.5 micrograms

Deficiency
weak muscles, nerve damage, fatigue

Toxicity
none known

VITAMIN B2 (RIBOFLAVIN)

Functions
energy release and cell repair

Best Food Sources
poultry, enriched breads, cereals and grains, as well as green leafy vegetables, organ meats, cheese, milk, and eggs

Requirements
1.2 to 1.8 milligrams

Deficiency
sore red tongue, dry flaky skin, cataracts

Toxicity
none known

NIACIN (NICOTINIC ACID)
Functions
allows cells to use fuel and oxygen
Best Food Sources
meat, fish, poultry, nuts, legumes, enriched cereals, whole grains
Requirements
13 to 20 milligrams
Deficiency
pellagra (symptoms may include dermatitis, diarrhea, and dementia)
Toxicity
in very high doses, flushed skin, possible liver damage, high blood sugar, and stomach ulcers

VITAMIN B6 (PYRIDOXINE)
Functions
assists in protein and red blood cell formation, helps produce anti-bodies and hormones.
Best Food Sources
meat, chicken, fish, organ meats, nuts, legumes, and whole grains
Requirements
1.5 to 2 milligrams
Deficiency
dermatitis, anemia, convulsions, and nausea
Toxicity
nerve damage

FOLATE (FOLACIN OR FOLIC ACID)
Functions
produces DNA and RNA to make cells, helps make red blood cells
Best Food Sources
dark green leafy vegetables, orange juice, dried beans, liver, whole grain breads, and cereals
Requirements
180 to 200 micrograms
Deficiency
increased risk of spina bifida in offspring, weakness, irritability, sore red tongue, diarrhea, weight loss, anemia
Toxicity
can mask B12 deficiency, which if untreated, can cause permanent nerve damage

121

VITAMIN B12 (COBALAMIN)

Functions

assists in DNA, RNA, and nerve formation, helps make red blood cells, facilitates energy metabolism

Best Food Sources

meat, poultry, fish, dairy products, and fortified foods

Requirements

2 micrograms

Deficiency

numb hands and feet, fatigue, anemia

Toxicity

none known

BIOTIN

Functions

assists in energy production

Best Food Sources

eggs, liver, dried beans, nuts, whole grains, cereals

Requirements

30 to 100 micrograms

Deficiency

loss of appetite, fatigue, dry skin, heart abnormalities, depression

Toxicity

none known

PANTOTHENIC ACID

Functions

assists in energy production

Best Food Sources

meat, poultry, fish, whole grains, legumes

Requirements

4 to 7 milligrams

Deficiency

numb hands and feet

Toxicity

diarrhea and water retention

MINERAL CHECKLIST

CALCIUM
Functions
   required for blood clotting, nerve, muscle, and cell membrane functions; builds bone and teeth, promotes enzyme reactions
Best Food Sources
   dairy products, green leafy vegetables, tofu, almonds, legumes
Requirements
   800 to 1200 milligrams
Deficiency
   increases risk for osteoporosis
Toxicity
   kidney stones and damage, constipation

PHOSPHORUS
Functions
   promotes bone, teeth, DNA, and RNA growth; assists in energy production
Best Food Sources
   meat, poultry, fish, eggs, legumes, nuts, breads
Requirements
   800 to 1200 milligrams
Deficiency
   bone loss, weakness, loss of appetite, pain
Toxicity
   decreases calcium levels in the blood leading to bone loss

MAGNESIUM
Functions
   component of bone and many enzymes; needed for energy production, muscle contractions, normal nerve and muscle cell functioning
Best Food Sources
   whole grains, legumes, nuts
Requirements
   280 to 400 milligrams
Deficiency
   muscle tremors, poor coordination, nausea, weakness, convulsions, poor appetite

Toxicity
nausea, low blood pressure, heart abnormalities, vomiting

CHROMIUM
Functions
allows body to use glucose
Best Food Sources
nuts, whole grains, meat
Requirements
50 to 200 micrograms
Deficiency
nerve damage and high blood sugar
Toxicity
none known

COPPER
Functions
facilitates energy production, component of enzymes, helps form hemoglobin and connective tissue
Best Food Sources
fruits, vegetables, nuts, seeds, legumes, liver
Requirements
1.5 to 3 milligrams
Deficiency
anemia
Toxicity
liver damage, coma, nausea, vomiting, and diarrhea

FLOURIDE
Functions
prevents tooth decay, strengthens bones
Best Food Sources
sardines, salmon, fluoridated water, and tea
Requirements
1.5 to 4 milligrams
Deficiency
tooth decay
Toxicity
brittle bones, stained or mottled teeth

IODINE
Functions
forms hormones that regulate the rate of energy usage
Best Food Sources
seafood, iodized table salt
Requirements
150 micrograms
Deficiency
enlarged thyroid, weight gain
Toxicity
enlarged thyroid

IRON
Functions
component of hemoglobin that carries oxygen to the cells
Best Food Sources
meat, poultry, fish, green leafy vegetables, dried fruits, legumes
Requirements
10 to 15 milligrams
Deficiency
infections, anemia, fatigue
Toxicity
poisonous to children; may lead to hemochromatosis

MANGANESE
Functions
a component of enzymes involved in energy and protein metabolism
Best Food Sources
whole grain products, tea, fruits, vegetables
Requirements
2 to 5 milligrams
Deficiency
rare
Toxicity
nerve damage

MOLYBDENUM
Functions
component of enzymes

Best Food Sources
organ meats, milk, legumes, and whole grains
Requirements
75 to 250 micrograms
Deficiency
rare
Toxicity
may interfere with copper use

SELENIUM
Functions
protects cells from damage, assists with cell growth
Best Food Sources
seafood, meats, grains, and seeds
Requirements
50 to 70 micrograms
Deficiency
may damage the heart
Toxicity
nerve damage, fatigue, irritability, nausea, vomiting, diarrhea, stomach pain

ZINC
Functions
necessary for wound healing, growth, reproduction, carbohydrate, protein, and alcohol metabolism, and for the production of DNA and RNA
Best Food Sources
meat, liver, eggs, dairy, whole grains, legumes, and oysters
Requirements
12 to 15 milligrams
Deficiency
loss of senses of taste and smell, loss of appetite, reduced resistance to infection, scaly skin, growth retardation
Toxicity
interferes with copper absorption and immune functioning, reduces good blood cholesterol (HDL), upsets stomach and may cause nausea and vomiting

SODIUM
Functions
regulates fluids, blood pressure, nerve and muscle function
Best Food Sources
processed foods, table salt
Requirements
a minimum of 500 milligrams
Deficiency
muscle cramps, dizziness, nausea, fatigue
Toxicity
may cause high blood pressure

POTASSIUM
Functions
fluid and mineral balance, blood pressure regulation, nerve and muscle function
Best Food Sources
fruits, vegetables, poultry, meat, fish
Requirements
a minimum of 2000 milligrams
Deficiency
abnormal heartbeat, muscle paralysis, weakness, lethargy
Toxicity
heart abnormalities

CHLORIDE
Functions
component of stomach acid, regulates fluid balance
Best Food Sources
table salt
Requirements
a minimum of 750 milligrams
Deficiency
growth failure, behavioral and learning problems, poor appetite
Toxicity
may cause high blood pressure

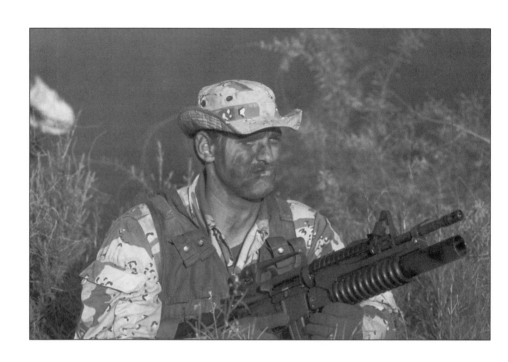

PREPARE YOURSELF
FOR THE SEALS

The following section has been excerpted from the Naval Special Warfare Web pages, which provide information to civilians and naval personnel interested in applying to BUD/S training. This excerpt focuses on physical fitness readiness. For complete SEALs and BUD/S information, contact your Navy recruiter.

The workouts on the following pages are designed for two groups: The Category I Workout is designed for individuals who have not recently, or have never, participated in a routine physical training (PT) program. The Category II Workout is designed for individuals who currently perform regular physical training. Athletes who participate in sports requiring a high degree of cardiovascular fitness—such as swimming, running, and wrestling—generally fall into Category II. The Category II workout is also appropriate for individuals who have completed the Category I program.

CATEGORY I WORKOUT

Category I is a progressive, nine-week program. Follow the workout to the best of your ability and you will be amazed at the progress you make.

Running
Most of the physical activities you will be required to perform during your six months of training at BUD/S involve running. Intense running

can lead to stress injuries of the lower extremities in trainees who arrive unprepared for it. Swimming, bicycling, and weight training will prepare you for some of the activities at BUD/S, but only running can prepare your legs for the rigors of the BUD/S program. You should also become accustomed to running in boots, a daily BUD/S activity. Select a lightweight boot such as Bates Lights.

The running distance goal of the Category I student is to work up to 16 miles per week. After you have achieved this goal, you will be ready to tackle the Category II goal of 30 miles per week.

Category I RUNNING SCHEDULE
Week 1 and 2 runs are at a 8:30 pace

	Mon.	Tues.	Wed.	Thurs.	Fri.	Total
Week 1	2		2		2	6
Week 2	2		2		2	6
Week 3	No running; high risk of stress fractures.					
Week 4	3		3		3	9
Week 5	2	3		4	2	11
Week 6	2	3		4	2	11
Week 7	4	4		5	3	16
Week 8	4	4		5	3	16
Week 9	4	4		5	3	16

Category I PHYSICAL TRAINING SCHEDULE
Monday, Wednesday, and Friday (Sets x Repetitions)

	Push-Ups	Sit-Ups	Pull-Ups
Week 1	4 x 15	4 x 20	3 x 3
Week 2	5 x 20	5 x 20	3 x 3
Week 3	5 x 25	5 x 25	3 x 4
Week 4	5 x 25	5 x 25	3 x 4
Week 5	6 x 25	6 x 25	2 x 8
Week 6	6 x 25	6 x 25	2 x 8
Week 7	6 x 30	6 x 30	2 x 10
Week 8	6 x 30	6 x 30	2 x 10
Week 9	6 x 30	6 x 30	3 x 10

Note: for best results, alternate exercise. Do a set of push-ups, then a set of sit-ups, followed by a set of pull-ups. Do not rest between sets.

Category I SWIMMING SCHEDULE
(Sidestroke with no fins, 4 to 5 days per week)

Week 1	Swim continuously for 15 minutes
Week 2	Swim continuously for 15 minutes
Week 3	Swim continuously for 20 minutes
Week 4	Swim continuously for 20 minutes
Week 5	Swim continuously for 25 minutes
Week 6	Swim continuously for 25 minutes
Week 7	Swim continuously for 30 minutes
Week 8	Swim continuously for 30 minutes
Week 9	Swim continuously for 35 minutes

Notes: If you have access to a pool, swim as often as possible. Your initial work-up goal is 4 to 5 days per week and 200 meters distance per session. Develop your sidestroke on both right and left sides. Try to swim 50 meters in one minute or less.

If you don't have access to a pool, ride a bicycle for twice as long as the recommended swim duration.

CATEGORY II WORKOUT

Do not attempt this workout schedule unless you can complete the Week 9 level of the Category I workout.

Running
Most of the physical activities you will be required to perform during your six months of training at BUD/S involve running. Intense running can lead to stress injuries of the lower extremities in trainees who arrive unprepared for it. Swimming, bicycling, and weight training will prepare you for some of the activities at BUD/S, but only running can prepare your legs for the rigors of the BUD/S program. You should also become accustomed to running in boots, a daily BUD/S activity. Select a lightweight boot such as Bates Lights.

Category II Running Schedule

	Mon.	Tues.	Wed.	Thurs.	Fri.	Total
Week 1	3	5	4	5	2	19
Week 2	3	5	4	5	2	19
Week 3	4	5	6	4	3	22
Week 4	4	5	6	4	3	22
Week 5	5	5	6	4	4	24
Week 6	5	6	6	6	4	27
Week 7	6	6	6	6	6	30

Notes: For Weeks 8 and beyond, you need not increase the distance of your runs. Instead, work on the speed of your 6-mile runs with an eye toward decreasing your time to 7:30 per mile or less.

If you wish to increase the distance of your runs, *do so gradually.* Do not increase your distance more than one mile per day for every week beyond Week 9.

Category II PHYSICAL TRAINING SCHEDULE
Monday, Wednesday, Friday (Sets x Repetitions)

	Push-Ups	Sit-Ups	Pull-Ups	Dips
Week 1	6 x 30	6 x 35	3 x 10	3 x 20
Week 2	6 x 30	6 x 35	3 x 10	3 x 20
Week 3	10 x 20	10 x 25	4 x 10	10 x 15
Week 4	10 x 20	10 x 25	4 x 10	10 x 15
Week 5	15 x 20	15 x 25	4 x 12	15 x 15
Week 6	20 x 20	20 x 25	5 x 12	20 x 15

Notes: These workouts are designed for long-distance muscle endurance. By performing high-repetition workouts, muscle fatigue will gradually take longer to develop.

For best results, alternate exercises each set to rest affected muscle groups for a short period.

Once you've met Categories I and II running and PT standards, you may vary your exercise program with the pyramid and swimming workouts below.

Category II SWIMMING SCHEDULE
(4 to 5 days per week)

Week 1	Swim continuously for 35 minutes
Week 2	Swim continuously for 35 minutes
Week 3	Swim continuously for 45 minutes
Week 4	Swim continuously for 45 minutes
Week 5	Swim continuously for 60 minutes
Week 6	Swim continuously for 75 minutes

Notes: When starting with fins, alternate swimming 1000 meters with fins and 1000 meters without. This will reduce initial stress on your foot muscles.

Your goal is to swim 50 meters in 45 seconds or less.

Pyramid Workouts
You can apply the pyramid method to any exercise. The object is to gradually build toward a target, then ease down to the level at the workout start. For instance, pull-ups, sit-ups, and push-ups can be alternated as in the previous workouts. But with the pyramid workout, choose a numerical goal and build up to it. In the sample table below, each number counts as a set. Work your way up and down the pyramid. The sample goal below is five sets.

Sample Pyramid Workout
Goal: 5 Sets

	Number of Repetitions
Pull-Ups	1, 2, 3, 4, 5, 4, 3, 2, 1
Push-Ups	(2x the no. of pull-ups): 2, 4, 6, 8, 10, 8, 6, 4, 2
Sit-Ups	(3x the no. of pull-ups): 3, 6, 9, 12, 15, 12, 9, 6, 3
Dips	1, 2, 3, 4, 5, 4, 3, 2, 1

Stretch PT
Since Monday, Wednesday, and Friday are devoted to PT, dedicate at least 20 minutes on Tuesday, Thursday, and Saturday to stretching. Always stretch for at least 15 minutes before beginning any workout. Simply stretching the previously worked muscles will make you more flexible and less likely to get injured.

Start your stretch PT at the top of your body and work downward. Stretch every muscle in your body from neck to calves, concentrating on your thighs, hamstrings, chest, back, and shoulders.

Stretch to tightness, not pain. Hold each stretch for 10 to 15 seconds. Do not bounce.

PHYSICAL FITNESS STANDARDS

The intense physical and mental conditioning required to become a SEAL begins with Basic Underwater Demolition/SEAL (BUD/S) training. During this six-month program, recruits are pushed to their physical and mental limits.

BUD/S students participate in challenging training and encounter on a daily basis opportunities to develop and test their stamina and leadership. BUD/S training is extremely thorough—both physically and mentally—but through adequate preparation and a positive attitude you can meet its challenges with confidence.

In each Phase of BUD/S (See *So You Want to be a Seal,* page 19), students must meet a series of physical fitness standards before proceeding to the next phase. Here are those standards.

First Phase

Task	Standard
50-meter underwater swim	Pass/fail
Underwater knot tying	Pass/fail
Drownproofing test (see page 135)	Pass/fail
Basic lifesaving test	Pass/fail
1200-meter pool swim with fins	45 minutes
1-mile bay swim with fins	50 minutes
1-mile ocean swim with fins	50 minutes
1.5-mile swim with fins	70 minutes
2-mile ocean swim with fins	95 minutes
Obstacle course	15 minutes
4-mile timed run	32 minutes

First Phase: Post-Hell Week

Task	Standard
2000-meter condition pool swim w/out fins	Completion
1.5-mile night bay swim with fins	Completion
2-mile ocean swim with fins	85 minutes
4-mile timed run in boots	32 minutes
Obstacle course	13 minutes

Second Phase

Task	Standard
2-mile ocean swim with fins	80 minutes
4-mile timed run in boots	31 minutes
Obstacle course	10.5 minutes
3.5-mile ocean swim with fins	Completion
5.5-mile ocean swim with fins	Completion

Third Phase

Task	Standard
4-mile timed run in boots	30 minutes
14-mile run	Completion
2-mile ocean swim with fins	75 minutes
Obstacle course	10 minutes

Required academic standards on written tests
Officers   80 percent or above
Enlisted   70 percent or above

Drownproofing
Objective: Demonstrate water confidence and competence under the most extreme conditions.

With hands tied behind back and feet bound, the student enters the water in the nine-foot-deep combat training tank and begins to bob for five minutes. Then he is instructed to remain on the surface and float for five minutes. After floating he then swims 100 meters. Upon completion of swim, the trainee then bobs again for two minutes, demonstrating underwater forward and reverse flips. Finally, the trainee successfully completes the evolution when he goes to the bottom of the tank, retrieves his mask with his teeth and then completes five bobs.

Successful completion of the drownproofing evolution illustrates to the staff and trainee both comfort and competency in the water. This drill is a leading indication of a student's ability to successfully complete the maritime aspect of BUD/S training.

Post-BUD/S Schools

BUD/S graduates receive three weeks of basic parachute training at Army Airborne School, Fort Benning, Georgia, prior to returning to the Naval Special Warfare Center for 15 weeks of SEAL Qualification Training (SQT).

After successfully completing SQT, qualified personnel are awarded a Naval Special Warfare designation Trident Insignia. They are then assigned to a SEAL Team. New combat swimmers serve the remainder of their first enlistment (2 1/2 to 3 years) in either an SDV or a SEAL Team. Upon reenlistment, the member may be ordered to the remainder of a five-year sea tour.

Navy corpsmen who complete BUD/S and Basic Airborne Training also attend two weeks of Special Operations Technician training at the Naval Special Warfare Center, Coronado. They also participate in an intense course of instruction in diving medicine and medical skills called 18-D (Special Operations Medical Sergeant Course). This is a 30-week course in which students receive training in treating burns, gunshot wounds, and trauma.

A broad range of advanced training opportunities is available. Advanced courses include: Sniper School, Dive Supervisor, language training, SEAL tactical communication, and many others. Shore duty opportunities are available in research and development, instructor duty, and overseas assignments.

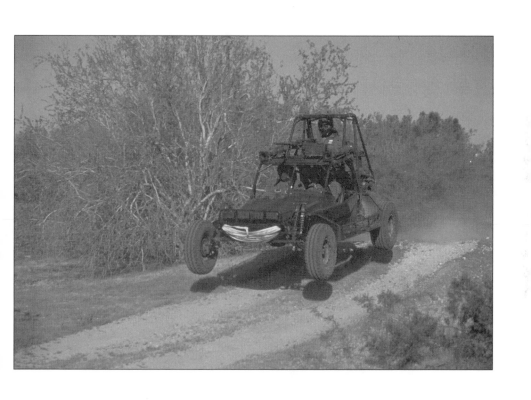

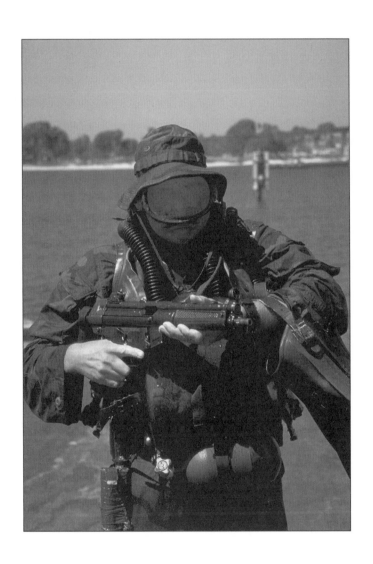

THE NAVY SEAL TOTAL BODY WORKOUT

The following workout schedules have been developed by the editors of Getfitnow.com Books. They incorporate the exercises you'll find in this book, and have been tailored to meet a variety of fitness levels. We hope that these guidelines will bring you to a level of fitness appropriate for your age and health.

Keep in mind it is *highly* recommended that you seek the advice of proper personnel who can design a training program suitable to your individual needs and that you consult a physician before commencing any new exercise program or before intensifying any existing exercise program. Also consider these important factors that may affect your fitness regimen:

Your age

Your recent physical fitness activities

Any medical conditions

Any health-related concern
(smoking, heavy alcohol consumption, weight issues)

The bottom line: Take your health seriously!

Level 1: Basic Training

Approximate time for the workout: 1 hour

An ideal starting point. Nice and easy. You'll get familiar with the exercises and within a few weeks, you'll feel a level of confidence to move to Level 2.

Level 2: Junior UDT

Approximate time for the workout: 1 hour

Moving up, you're still getting used to a regular fitness routine. You're introduced to a variety of pull-up variations and your ab workout is intensified. Running or swimming is required in the cardio portion of your workout.

Level 3: Future Seal

Approximate time for the workout: 1 1/2 hours

It's *almost* time to take the training wheels off. At this level you'll add some push-up variations and get acquainted with rope climbing. If you have trouble finding a rope to climb, well, look harder! Rope climbing is a phenomenal way to build upper body strength. Warm-ups now include running, not walking.

Level 4: Fit as a Frogman

Approximate time for the workout: 2 hours

Solid, heavy-duty PT. If you achieve this level of fitness, you're going to be in fantastic shape. Frogmen love the water, so you might want to alternate swimming and running as your cardio workouts. Learn the proper swim strokes: Check out *The Complete Guide to Navy SEAL Fitness* by Stewart Smith for a thorough presentation of swimming in the Navy SEALs.

Level 5: Braving BUD/S

Approximate time for the workout: 2 hours

This is a combination of PT exercises you'll find the BUD/S candidates performing at the Naval Special Warfare Center. It's no-holds-barred as you punch through a grinding PT with the best of them. Too easy? Add sets, increase reps. Still too easy? Check out the recruiting information and apply for BUD/S. Once there, your instructors will find a variety of ways to challenge you physically and mentally.

To determine the level at which you should begin, use the following suggested guidelines:

Level	1	2	3	4	5
Push-Ups (in 2 min.)	1-10	11-20	21-30	31-50	51+
Pull-Ups (max)	0-3	4-9	10-15	16-25	26+
Sit-Ups (in 2 min.)	5-15	16-25	26-40	41-60	61+
Running (1 mile)	Can't do it	12:00	10:00	9:00	8:00
Swimming (.25 mile)	Can't do it	20:00	15:00	12:00	10:00

There are two ways to choose a starting category for yourself. One way is to test your ability in each exercise and start at the level of your "worst" performance. So, for example, if you can do 20 push-ups but can't run a mile, start at Level 1. If you can do 50 sit-ups but only 6 pull-ups, start at Level 2. You could also mix levels, for instance, doing the number of sit-ups from Level 3 but the number of pull-ups from Level 2. No matter which method you use to choose a starting level, stick with that level for at least 4 weeks. If it becomes too easy (you'll know when), increase the number of reps per exercise. If it's still too easy, add another set. Whatever you do, stick with the schedule!

Check out our Web site: www.getfitnow.com, and our discussion area about this and other workouts. You can ask questions, get feedback, and find out about others' experiences with the Navy SEAL Workout.

WEEKLY WORKOUT SCHEDULE

	Sunday	Monday	Tuesday	Wednesday	Thursday	Friday	Saturday
	OFF	Warm-up/ Stretch	Warm-up/ Stretch	Warm-up/ Stretch	Warm-up/ Stretch	Warm-up/ Stretch	Warm-up/ Stretch
		Upper Body PT Pull-up PT	Lower Body PT	Upper Body PT Pull-up PT	Lower Body PT	Upper Body PT Pull-up PT	
		Abs PT	Abs PT	Abs PT	Abs PT	Abs PT	
		Body Builders	Body Builders	Body Builders	Body Builders	Body Builders	
		Cardio	Cardio	Cardio	Cardio	Cardio	
		Rope Climb	Rope Climb	Rope Climb	Rope Climb	Rope Climb	Rope Climb

RUN	
Level	Miles
1	1
2	2
3	3
4	4
5	5
6	6

Note: Stick with your workout level for 4 weeks. If it gets too easy, increase the number of reps per exercise. If it's still too easy, add another set.

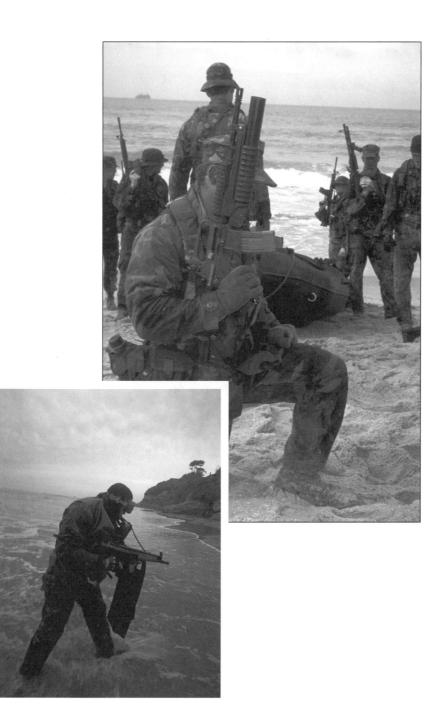

LEVEL 1

WARM UP

Walk/Jog	15 min.

STRETCH

Hurdler or Modified Hurdler	Left and Right (L/R) 30 sec.
Sitting Head to Knee	30 sec.
Back Rollers (optional)	30 sec.
Butterfly Stretch	30 sec.
Groin Stretch	30 sec.
Ilio Tibial Band (ITB) Stretch	L/R 30 sec.
Swimmer Stretch	30 sec.
Triceps Stretch	L/R 15 sec.
Press-Press-Fling	10
Up, Back and Over	10
Trunk Rotations	4
Trunk Bending Fore and Aft	5

UPPER BODY

Regular Push-Ups	10
Arm Haulers	10

ABDOMINALS

Sit-Ups	10
Leg Levers	10
Atomic Sit-Ups	5
Back Flutter Kicks	10
Crunches—Heel in Close	10
Crunches—Legs Up	10
Cross-Legs Sit-Ups	L/R 6
Sitting Flutter Kick*	5
Sitting Knee Benders*	5
Scissors*	10
Sitting Bicycles*	10
Neck Rotations*	L/R 15, Up and Down (U/D) 20

LEVEL 1

LOWER BODY

Lunges	10
Squat Leaps	5

PULL-UPS

Pull-Ups, Regular Grip	max
Pull-Ups, Reverse Grip	max
Dips	max

CARDIO

Treadmill: Walking	1.5 mi.
Or	
Swimming	.25 mi.

OTHER

Eight-Count Body Builder	5

* These exercises are optional or substitutes.

LEVEL 2

WARM UP

Walk/Jog   15 min.

STRETCH

Hurdler or Modified Hurdler	Left and Right (L/R) 30 sec.
Sitting Head to Knee	30 sec.
Back Rollers (optional)	30 sec.
Butterfly Stretch	30 sec.
Groin Stretch	30 sec.
ITB Stretch	L/R 30 sec.
Swimmer Stretch	30 sec.
Triceps Stretch	L/R 15 sec.
Press-Press-Fling	10
Up, Back and Over	10
Trunk Rotations	4
Trunk Bending Fore and Aft	5

UPPER BODY

Regular Push-Ups	10 x 2
Arm Haulers	15

ABDOMINALS

Sit-Ups	25
Leg Levers	25
Atomic Sit-Ups	10
Back Flutter Kicks	20
Crunches—Heel in Close	10 x 2
Crunches—Legs Up	10 x 2
Cross-Legs Sit-Ups	L/R 12
Sitting Flutter Kick*	10
Sitting Knee Benders*	10
Scissors*	20
Sitting Bicycles*	20
Neck Rotations*	L/R 15, U/D 20

LEVEL 2

LOWER BODY

Lunges	15
Squat Leaps	10
Side Lunge	5

PULL-UPS

Pull-Ups, Regular Grip	max x 2
Pull-Ups, Wide Grip	max
Pull-Ups, Reverse Grip	max x 2
Pull-Ups, Close Grip	max
Cliffhangers	max
Dips	max x 2

CARDIO

Treadmill: Running	1 mi.
Or	
Swimming	.50 mi.

OTHER

Eight-Count Body Builder	10

* These exercises are optional or substitutes.

LEVEL 3

WARM UP

Running   1 mi.

STRETCH

Hurdler or Modified Hurdler	Left and Right (L/R) 30 sec.
Sitting Head to Knee	30 sec.
Back Rollers (optional)	30 sec.
Butterfly Stretch	30 sec.
Groin Stretch	30 sec.
ITB Stretch	L/R 30 sec.
Swimmer Stretch	30 sec.
Triceps Stretch	L/R 15 sec.
Press-Press-Fling	10
Up, Back and Over	10
Trunk Rotations	4
Trunk Bending Fore and Aft	5

UPPER BODY

Regular Push-Ups	15 x 2
Triceps Push-Ups	7 x 2
Dive Bomber Push-Ups	10 x 2
Arm Haulers	20

ABDOMINALS

Sit-Ups	25 x 2
Leg Levers	25 x 2
Atomic Sit-Ups	10 x 2
Back Flutter Kicks	20 x 2
Crunches—Heel in Close	20 x 2
Extended Leg Crunches	20 x 2
Cross-Legs Sit-Ups	L/R 12 x 2
Sitting Flutter Kick*	10 x 2
Sitting Knee Benders*	10 x 2
Scissors*	20 x 2

LEVEL 3

ABDOMINALS (cont'd)

Sitting Bicycles*	20 x 2
Neck Rotations*	L/R 15, U/D 20

LOWER BODY

Lunges	20
Squat Leaps	15
Side Lunge	10
Star Jumpers	5

PULL-UPS

Pull-Ups, Regular Grip	4 x 2
Pull-Ups, Wide Grip	4 x 2
Pull-Ups, Reverse Grip	4 x 2
Pull-Ups, Close Grip	4 x 2
Cliffhangers	4 x 2
Dips	5 x 2

CARDIO

Treadmill: Running	2 mi.
Or	
Swimming	.75 mi.

OTHER

Rope Climb	30 ft. x 1
Eight-Count Body Builder	15

* These exercises are optional or substitutes.

LEVEL 4

WARM UP

Running	1.5 mi.

STRETCH

Hurdler or Modified Hurdler	Left and Right (L/R) 30 sec.
Sitting Head to Knee	30 sec.
Back Rollers (optional)	30 sec.
Butterfly Stretch	30 sec.
Groin Stretch	30 sec.
ITB Stretch	L/R 30 sec.
Swimmer Stretch	30 sec.
Triceps Stretch	L/R 15 sec.
Press-Press-Fling	10
Up, Back and Over	10
Trunk Rotations	4
Trunk Bending Fore and Aft	5

UPPER BODY

Regular Push-Ups	20 x 2
Triceps Push-Ups	10 x 2
Dive Bomber Push-Ups	15 x 2
Arm Haulers	25

ABDOMINALS

Sit-Ups	35 x 2
Leg Levers	35 x 2
Atomic Sit-Ups	15 x 2
Back Flutter Kicks*	30 x 2
Crunches—Heel in Close*	30 x 2
Extended Leg Crunches*	30 x 2
Cross-Legs Sit-Ups*	L/R 18 x 2
Sitting Flutter Kick*	15 x 2
Sitting Knee Benders*	15 x 2
Scissors*	30 x 2

LEVEL 4

ABDOMINALS (cont'd)

Sitting Bicycles*	30 x 2
Neck Rotations*	L/R 15, U/D 20

LOWER BODY

Lunges	25
Squat Leaps	20
Side Lunge	15
Star Jumpers	10

PULL-UPS

Pull-Ups, Regular Grip	5 x 2
Pull-Ups, Wide Grip	5 x 2
Pull-Ups, Reverse Grip	5 x 2
Pull-Ups, Close Grip	5 x 2
Cliffhangers	5 x 2
Dip	10 x 3

CARDIO

Treadmill: Running	3 mi.
Or	
Swimming (miles)	1 mi.

OTHER

Rope Climb	30 ft. x 2
Eight-Count Body Builder	20

* These exercises are optional or substitutes.

LEVEL 5

WARM UP

Running	2 mi.

STRETCH

Hurdler or Modified Hurdler	Left and Right (L/R) 30 sec.
Sitting Head to Knee	30 sec.
Back Rollers (optional)	30 sec.
Butterfly Stretch	30 sec.
Groin Stretch	30 sec.
ITB Stretch	L/R 30 sec.
Swimmer Stretch	30 sec.
Triceps Stretch	L/R 15 sec.
Press-Press-Fling	10
Up, Back and Over	10
Trunk Rotations	4
Trunk Bending Fore and Aft	5

UPPER BODY

Regular Push-Ups	20 x 3
Triceps Push-Ups	10 x 3
Dive Bomber Push-Ups	15 x 3
Arm Haulers	30

ABDOMINALS

Sit-Ups	50 x 2
Leg Levers	50 x 2
Atomic Sit-Ups	20 x 2
Back Flutter Kicks	40 x 2
Crunches—Heel in Close	40 x 2
Extended Leg Crunches	40 x 2
Cross-Legs Sit-Ups	L/R 25 x 2
Sitting Flutter Kicks*	20 x 2
Sitting Knee Benders*	20 x 2
Scissors*	40 x 2

LEVEL 5

ABDOMINALS (cont'd)

Sitting Bicycles*	40 x 2
Neck Rotations*	L/R 15, U/D 20

LOWER BODY

Lunges	30
Squat Leaps	25
Side Lunge	20
Star Jumpers	15

PULL-UPS

Pull-Ups, Regular Grip	6 x 2
Pull-Ups, Wide Grip	6 x 2
Pull-Ups, Reverse Grip	6 x 22
Pull-up Close	6 x 2
Cliffhangers	6 x 2
Dips	15 x 3

CARDIO

Treadmill: Running	4 mi.
Or	
Swimming	1.5 mi.

OTHER

Rope Climb	30 ft. x 3
Eight-Count Body Builder	25

* These exercises are optional or substitutes.

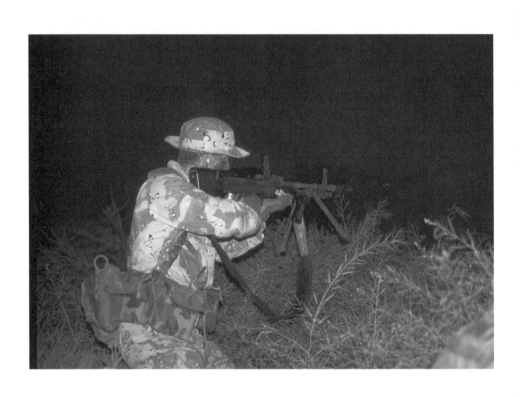

HOW TO BECOME A NAVY SEAL

The Navy SEALs have a long, proud history. And today the SEALs are active around the world, including in Afghanistan, where they play an integral part in Operation Enduring Freedom. They're on the front lines, searching caves for intelligence, calling in air strikes, and—most dangerous of all—fighting in combat, aka direct-action missions. These elite forces uncovered a vast network of al-Qaeda caves in which caches of weapons and intelligence documents were found. Those documents and the SEALs work is helping to unravel the story of the al-Qaeda terrorist network.

For more information about becoming a Navy SEAL, speak with your local Navy recruiter or contact one of the following sources.

SEAL Recruiters

SEAL recruiters are active-duty SEALs assigned to recruiting billets of the U.S. Navy. Although they have particular knowledge about Naval Special Warfare, they are often employed as recruiters for the Navy as a whole, not just the SEAL community. They are stationed in various parts of the country, and if stationed near you, can be an invaluable resource in helping you to secure a SEAL Challenge contract or develop a physical fitness program to prepare you for BUD/S.

ISC(SEAL) Cary Cooley
BMCS(SEAL) Frank Hoagland
Aurora, Colo.
Steubenville, O.H.
Phone: 303-937-9145
Phone: 740-282-3435
Email: caryc_brew@hotmail.com
Email: ohbuki@1st.net

HM1(SEAL) Jared Holforty
Sandy, Utah
Phone: 801-572-4470
Email: 83748100@cnrc.navy.mil

GM2(SEAL) Matt Kelm
Edmond, Okla.
Phone: (405) 715-3566
Email: seal_dal@cnrc.navy.mil

OS1 (SEAL) Buddy Ketchum
Southbridge, Mass.
Phone: 508-764-4512
Email: frogat5@hotmail.com

SEAL Motivators

West Coast SEAL Motivator

BMC(SEAL) Mike Getka
San Diego, Calif.
Phone: (619) 437-5009
Email: recruiting@navsoc.navy.mil

East Coast SEAL Motivator

HM1(SEAL) Mark Ridgeway
Norfolk, Va.
Phone: (757) 462-4128
Email: ridgewaym@
grp2.nswlant.navy.mil

Dive Motivator

(For enlisted and delayed entry
personnel)
Great Lakes, Ill.
Phone: (847) 688-4643

SEAL and SWCC motivators are active-duty SEALs and SWCC assigned to Naval Special Warfare Command and stationed in fleet concentration areas of Norfolk, Virginia, and San Diego, California. Their role is to disseminate information about NSW to interested applicants.

Navy SEAL Challenge Contract

The SEAL Challenge Contract is the *only* enlistment contract that guarantees you an opportunity to compete for a place at BUD/S. Here's a sample.

Enlistment Guarantees

Frogman, Joe Jumpin   123-45-6789
NAME (LAST, FIRST, MIDDLE, JR., ETC.)   SSN

1. ACKNOWLEDGEMENT: In connection with my enlistment into the United States Navy I hereby acknowledge that:

    a. I am enlisting into the U.S. Navy for an active duty period of 4 years. I am enlisting with the following guarantees and understanding:

        (1) Upon enlistment, I will be enlisted under the provisions of CNRC Instruction 1130.8, option or options as indicated below:

        Option (1) SEAL Challenge Program/Applicable class "A" school
        Option (2) Enlistment Bonus (amount per latest EB message).
        Option (3) NA.
        Option (4) NA.

2. I understand that I must be fully qualified at all times throughout my obligated service for all security, professional, military, physical, psychological and academic requirements of the options guaranteed in section 1a (1) and that my eligibility will be rechecked during recruit training and periodically throughout my enlistment.

3. The Navy will enroll me in the training specified above. If during the periodic reviews of my eligibility, I am found no longer eligible for the options listed in 1a(1) above because of information I provided in my enlistment application; because of a physical or psychological disqualification, or because of some reason that is not due to my fault, negligence, or conduct, I may only choose one of the following options:

    a. Reassignment to an "A" school for which I am qualified and a vacancy exists, or

    b. Navy apprentice training for which I am qualified and a vacancy exists.

In any event, the Navy may, at its option, choose to discharge me.

4. If I am not enrolled in the training guarantee specified in section 1a(1) above because of some reason that is due to my fault, negligence or conduct or if I am disenrolled from it for any other reason not specified in paragraph 3, then I lose that guarantee and at the Navy's option remain subject to continued naval service. I also understand:

a. If I am retained, I may be required to serve the rest of my enlistment. If given accelerated advancement, post-apprentice training, or an enlistment/reenlistment bonus, I may incur additional service as required by regulation.

b. The Navy may, at its option, discharge me in accordance with law and regulation.

5. I certify that I have read and received a copy of the Classifier Rating/Program Fact Sheet for the Rating/Program for which I am enlisting, and the Statement of Understandings required for Options (1). (2).

I understand the obligations for the Options and training that I will receive

_____

(applicant's initials)

_____   _____

(Signature of Enlisting Officer)/Date   (Signature of Enlistee)/Date

Annex A to DD Form 4 dated 5 APR 91.
NAVCRUIT 1133/52 (Rev. 10-94)

UDT-SEAL MUSEUM

The Underwater Demolition Teams—better known as Frogmen—and the SEAL Teams, along with the Scouts, Raiders, and the Naval Combat Demolition Units, have a history shrouded in secrecy. The UDT-SEAL Museum is the only museum in the world dedicated exclusively to these elite fighting men.

The SEALs are one of our country's most highly decorated combat units, earning three Medals of Honor, numerous Navy Crosses, Legions of Merit, Silver Stars, and hundreds of other medals.

The UDT-SEAL Museum is on the original training ground of the U.S. Navy Frogmen in Fort Pierce, Florida, where these unique underwater warriors were born in May 1943.

Now's the time to joint the UDT-SEAL Museum Association! Help preserve the heritage of the Underwater Demolition Teams and the SEAL Teams of the U.S. Navy! Begin or renew a membership, volunteer, or give a gift membership. For more information about the UDT-SEAL Museum, write, call, visit, or email:

UDT-SEAL Museum
3300 North A1A
North Hutchinson Island
Fort Pierce, FL 34949-8520
Phone (561) 595-5845 Fax (561) 595-5847
Web site: http://www.udt-seal.org/museum.html
Email: museumoffice@aol.com

Hours of Operation
Monday (January 1-May 1 only): 10:00 A.M. to 4:00 P.M.
Tuesday through Saturday: 10:00 A.M. to 4:00 P.M.
Sunday: Noon to 4:00 P.M.
Admission: Adults: $4; Children 6 to 12: $1.50, Pre-Schoolers: Free

ABOUT THE AUTHORS

Andrew Flach is a recognized authority on the subjects of fitness, diet and exercise. He is certified by the American Council on Exercise (ACE) as a Lifestyle and Weight Management Consultant. His unique brand of fitness synthesizes a wide variety of techniques—including military fitness, nutritionists' research, functional training, and the Surgeon General's guidelines—into comprehensive, practical, and easy-to-follow diet and fitness programs. His books are widely used both by civilians and the military to maintain the highest possible levels of physical fitness. His recent books include *Combat Fat!, The Official United States Naval Academy Workout* and *The Official United States Navy SEAL Workout*.

Peter Field Peck is one of the leading sports/fitness photojournalists in the United States. His photos have appeared in numerous books, magazines, and newspapers, including the *New York Post*, *Time*, and *USA Today*. He lives in Queens, New York.

THE COMPLETE GUIDE TO NAVY SEAL FITNESS

REVISED EDITION

By Stewart Smith, USN (SEAL)

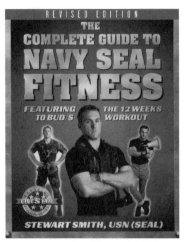

The *Official Navy SEAL Workout* gave you a glimpse into the world of the SEALs. Now follow the only workout that will get you into the SEALs!

It takes optimal fitness to swim 6 miles, run 15 miles, and perform over 150 pull-ups, 400 pushups, and 400 sit-ups in one day. More important, it takes determination to stick with it to the end. Follow and finish this workout and you'll be in the best physical shape of your life!

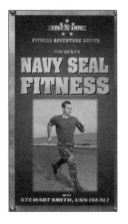

This revised edition brings you: expanded information about what it takes to be a Navy SEAL, including recruitment and preparation; insider's tips to negotiating the famous Navy SEAL obstacle course; new and improved chapters on swimming, running, and nutrition.

The Complete Guide to Navy Seal Fitness is an advanced exercise program that teaches running, swimming, rope climbing, stretching, and exercise techniques in one book. It will get you ready for any military training or physical challenge in the world. Train with the world's fittest and strongest: the US Navy SEALs!

Fully illustrated...packed with photos...just $15.95!

Available in bookstores or direct from the publisher:
Toll-Free Orders 1-800-906-1234
Order online at www.getfitnow.com

THE NAVY SEAL NUTRITION GUIDE

Patricia A. Deuster, PhD, Anita Singh, PhD, and Pierrre A. Pelletier, ENS, MC, USNR

and

THE NAVY SEAL PHYSICAL FITNESS GUIDE

Edited by Patricia A. Deuster, PhD

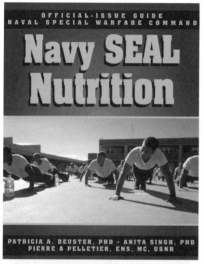

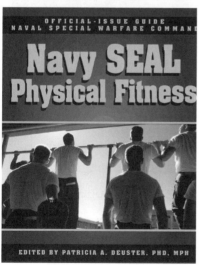

**Eat like a Navy SEAL.
Train like a Navy SEAL.**

Your Navy SEAL library won't be complete without **The Navy SEAL Nutrition Guide** and **The Navy SEAL Physical Fitness Guide**—both official publications of the United States Navy. These are the guides that keep SEALs fit, healthy, and ready for action. Written by some of the most knowledgeable fitness and nutrition specialists, medical doctors, and physiologists around, these guides cover anything and everything you need to stay in combat-ready shape.

**Official...essential...
authentic...just $19.95 each!**

Available in bookstores or direct from the publisher:

Toll-Free Orders 1-800-906-1234

Order online at www.getfitnow.com

THE UNITED STATES MARINE CORPS WORKOUT

Researched by Andrew Flach
Photographed by Peter Field Peck

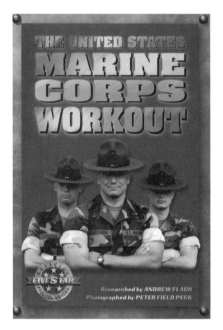

See the leathernecks in action!

For this fitness adventure, you'll join Charlie Company at the Officer's Candidate School at the U.S. Marine Corps Base in Quantico, Virginia. You'll discover training techniques you've never seen before. These are rugged workouts for rugged souls. You want to get fit? Tell it to the Marines!

You'll learn:

- **How to improve your upper and lower body and abdominal strength**
- **How the Marines prepare mentally for their grueling workouts**
- **Traditions and customs of the Marines • Total body workouts**
- **Plus dozens of powerful photographs!**

Whether you want to be a Marine or just be as tough as one, this is one book you don't want to miss. *Semper Fi!*

Intense workouts...great photos...just $14.95!

Available in bookstores or direct from the publisher:
Toll-Free Orders 1-800-906-1234
Order online at www.getfitnow.com

THE OFFICIAL UNITED STATES NAVAL ACADEMY WORKOUT

Researched by Andrew Flach
Photographed by Peter Field Peck

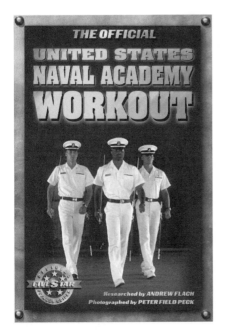

"The United States Naval Academy emphasizes the importance of being physically fit and prepared for stress, because the duty of Navy and Marine Corps officers often require long, strenuous hours in difficult situations."

The United States Naval Academy has spent decades developing a physical fitness program that maximizes fitness potential. This program can be done by anyone, anywhere. Now, for the first time, you can use this 6-week program to achieve total physical excellence.

Join Midshipmen Quintin Jones and Julia Mason as they lead you through a normal day's P.E.P. (Physical Education Program): stretches, upper and lower body PT, abdominal exercises, and more. Along the way, you'll learn dozens of fascinating facts about The United States Naval Academy—its history, traditions, training, and way of life. Don't miss your chance to work out with the future officers of the United States Navy. Start your Physical Education Program today!

Packed with photos...indispensible advice...just $14.95!

Available in bookstores or direct from the publisher:
Toll-Free Orders 1-800-906-1234
Order online at www.getfitnow.com

THE OFFICIAL UNITED STATES AIR FORCE ELITE WORKOUT

Researched by Andrew Flach

Photographed by Peter Field Peck

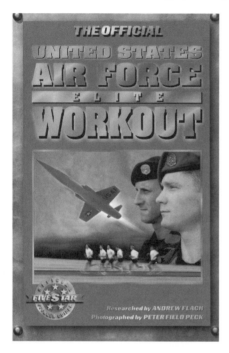

You know the SEALs . . . now meet their blood brothers!

Known as the PJs and the CCTs, the pararescuemen and combat control technicians are the elite forces of the United States Air Force. PJs—whose motto is *that others may live*—routinely go in harm's way to rescue downed pilots and crewmembers.

First There is the credo of the CCTs, whose job it is to enter hostile territory and establish safe landing sites for arriving forces. Their self-sacrificing efforts are heroic. Their training is intense, exciting, and before this book, little known. Now for the very first time, their powerful training techniques are brought to light in this profusely illustrated and documented book. You'll learn about stretching, weight-training, running, swimming, rope climbing, and more!

Fully illustrated...packed with information...just $14.95!

Available in bookstores or direct from the publisher:

Toll-Free Orders 1-800-906-1234

Order online at www.getfitnow.com